Cataract - An Update on Clinical and Surgical Management

*Edited by Salvatore Di Lauro,
David Jose Galarreta Mira
and Sara Crespo Millas*

Published in London, United Kingdom

Cataract - An Update on Clinical and Surgical Management
http://dx.doi.org/10.5772/intechopen.1000236
Edited by Salvatore Di Lauro, David Jose Galarreta Mira and Sara Crespo Millas

Contributors
Sara Crespo Millas, Salvatore Di Lauro, David Galarreta Mira, Brian A. Bird, Albert Y. Cheung, John D. Sheppard, Kenneth Gek-Jin Ooi, King Fai Calvin Leung, Jessica Xiong, Pauline Khoo, Stephanie Louise Watson, Ezgi Karataş, Canan Aslı Utine, Mohamed Al-Abri, Washoo Mal, Nawal Al-Fadhil

First published in London, United Kingdom, 2023 by IntechOpen
IntechOpen is the global imprint of INTECHOPEN LIMITED, registered in England and Wales, registration number: 11086078, 5 Princes Gate Court, London, SW7 2QJ, United Kingdom

British Library Cataloguing-in-Publication Data
A catalogue record for this book is available from the British Library

Additional hard and PDF copies can be obtained from orders@intechopen.com

Cataract - An Update on Clinical and Surgical Management
Edited by Salvatore Di Lauro, David Jose Galarreta Mira and Sara Crespo Millas
p. cm.
Print ISBN 978-1-83769-652-9
Online ISBN 978-1-83769-651-2
eBook (PDF) ISBN 978-1-83769-653-6

Meet the editors

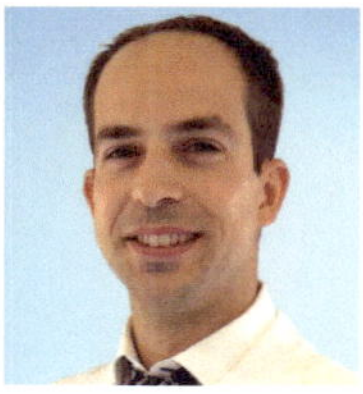

Salvatore Di Lauro graduated in medicine and surgery from the University of Naples "Federico II," Italy, in 2009. He obtained a master's degree in vitreo-retina from the University of Valladolid, Spain, becoming a specialist in ophthalmology. He is a fellow of the European Board of Ophthalmology and has been an Honorific Collaborator of the University of Valladolid. He is an active researcher in retinal and ocular surface diseases, participating as investigator and study coordinator in numerous clinical trials, and has published several papers and book chapters. He is part of the REPRISE database of expert reviewers created by the Italian Ministry of Education, Universities, and Research.

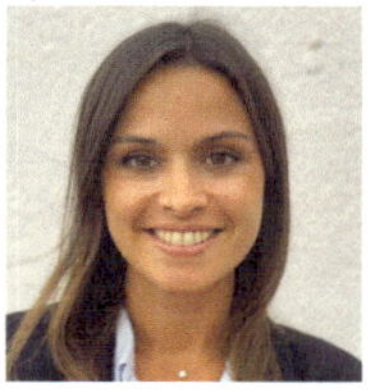

Sara Crespo Millas graduated in medicine and surgery from the Autonomous University of Madrid, Spain, receiving a master's degree in vitreo-retina from the University of Valladolid, Spain, and the title of specialist in ophthalmology. She is a researcher in retinal and ocular surface diseases, participating as an investigator in various clinical trials, and has presented at several recent international congresses.

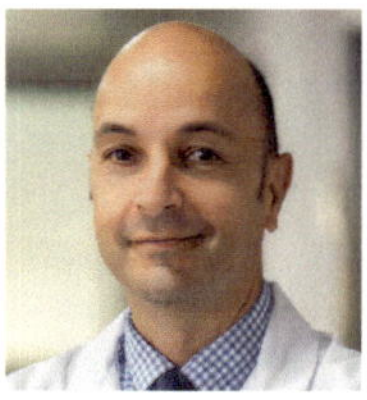

David Galarreta Mira graduated in medicine and surgery from the University of Navarra, Spain, and obtained his Ph.D. in Medicine and Surgery from the University of Valladolid, Spain. He is an associate researcher at the Recognized Research Group (GIR) of Optical Diagnostic Techniques (TOD) at the University of Valladolid, and an associate researcher in the Results-Oriented Cooperative Research Networks in Health (RICORS). He has been the principal investigator for many clinical trials and competitive projects. He is also the author of multiple publications and book chapters.

Contents

Preface **IX**

Chapter 1 **1**
Antiseptic and Antibiotic Prophylaxis for Cataract Surgery
by Sara Crespo Millas, Salvatore Di Lauro and David Galarreta Mira

Chapter 2 **9**
Corneal Disease and Its Impact on Cataract Surgery
by Brian A. Bird, Albert Y. Cheung and John D. Sheppard

Chapter 3 **35**
Cataract Surgery and Dry Eye
by Kenneth Gek-Jin Ooi, King Fai Calvin Leung, Jessica Xiong, Pauline Khoo and Stephanie Louise Watson

Chapter 4 **63**
Evolution of Biometric Formulas and Intraocular Lens Selection in Challenging Cases
by Ezgi Karataş and Canan Aslı Utine

Chapter 5 **91**
Cataract Surgery Complications: *Vitreo-Retina Perspectives*
by Mohamed Al-Abri, Washoo Mal and Nawal Al-Fadhil

Preface

Ophthalmology is continuously evolving, with new imaging techniques, diagnostic tools, and therapeutic options. Cataract surgery is still the most performed surgery worldwide. The surgery is continuously evolving and there are ongoing efforts to make it safer with adequate infectious prophylaxis, and more precise with advanced intraocular lens (IOL) calculation. In this sense, the ocular surface is an important factor and must always be carefully analyzed. Complications may occur during and after cataract surgery, thus it is important to manage them correctly to obtain the best result.

This book is a collection of review chapters from international experts addressing recent innovations in cataract surgery.

Our special thanks go to Zrinka Tomicic at IntechOpen for her excellent work during the preparation of this book.

Salvatore Di Lauro MD, FEBO
University Clinical Hospital of Valladolid,
Ophthalmology Department,
Valladolid, Spain

Recoletas Ophthalmological Institute,
Vitreo-Retinal Department,
Valladolid, Spain

Sara Crespo Millas, MD
University Clinical Hospital of Valladolid,
Ophthalmology Department,
Valladolid, Spain

David Galarreta Mira, Ph.D., MD
University Clinical Hospital of Valladolid,
Ophthalmology Department,
Valladolid, Spain

Recoletas Ophthalmological Institute,
Ocular Surface Department,
Valladolid, Spain

Chapter 1

Antiseptic and Antibiotic Prophylaxis for Cataract Surgery

Sara Crespo Millas, Salvatore Di Lauro and David Galarreta Mira

Abstract

Prophylaxis for eye infections is important to avoid catastrophic consequences such as infectious endophthalmitis. There are different options as prophylaxis in cataract surgery. Prophylaxis with antiseptics is more and more important in ocular surgery and possesses several advantages compared to antibiotic prophylaxis. Povidone-iodine (PVI) 5% in the conjunctival sac and PVI 10% on periocular skin for 3 minutes is recommended prior to any cataract surgery to reduce the risk of postoperative endophthalmitis. Intracameral cefuroxime (1 mg/0.1 ml) at the end of the surgery is also useful in reducing the risk of infectious endophthalmitis. Nevertheless, there is no scientific evidence supporting the use of topical antibiotics in the postoperative period.

Keywords: cataract surgery, prophylaxis, antiseptic, antibiotic, endophthalmitis

1. Introduction

Infectious endophthalmitis after cataract surgery is an uncommon but devastating complication [1–4]. Infectious prophylaxis is essential in any eye surgery to prevent the infectious endophthalmitis. There are two forms of prophylaxis: antiseptic and antibiotic prophylaxis. The correct use of antibiotics is critical to avoid any unnecessary microorganism resistance able to reduce the already limited therapeutic options available to treat eye infections. Prophylaxis with antiseptics is more and more important in ocular surgery and possesses several advantages compared to antibiotic prophylaxis.

2. Antiseptics

The ideal antiseptic may have a wide spectrum of antimicrobial activity, including pathogens in biofilms, limited inactivation by organic compounds, good penetration including in the necrotic tissue with limited systemic absorption, without risk of acquired microbial resistance, good local and systemic tolerance, ability to aid cicatrization, may be easy to use and cheap [5, 6].

Povidone-iodine (PVI) is the most widely used antiseptic for ocular surgery. The PVI is a disinfectant and antiseptic of intermediate level [5, 6]. It is used in different concentrations (between 0.1 and 10%) depending on the country, but the most frequent concentrations are 5% in the conjunctival sac and 10% in periocular skin [5, 6].

The concentration of free iodine is already maximum with PVI 0.01–1%, obtaining minimum bactericide time. Nevertheless, free iodine is inactivated by the interaction with bacteria and organic compounds and with those concentrations it is necessary to repeat the PVI administration to maintain the bactericide effect [6]. PVI 2.5–10% generates enough free iodine reserve concentration to avoid the need for repeated administrations with a contact time of 3 minutes [1, 6].

PVI has well-known toxicity on the corneal epithelium and is directly related to the concentration and contact time [6]. PVI is toxic in vitro for epithelial cells, fibroblasts and endothelial cells in animal models. Nevertheless, repeated exposure during cataract surgery at 0.25% concentration is not toxic for the endothelium [6]. The application of PVI 5% is also safe for the endothelium [6].

Allergic reactions to PVI are rare and frequently reported by the patient and not confirmed [7]. Most frequently, contact dermatitis appears and is incorrectly classified as an allergy. There are no reports of anaphylactic reactions after topical ophthalmic use of PVI [8]. Iodine contrast allergy does not mean allergy to PVI [9]. In cases of real PVI allergy, there are alternative antiseptics available such as chlorhexidine.

Chlorhexidine is a cationic biguanide able to damage the bacterial cellular wall and cytoplasm. It is considered as a low-level disinfectant with lower microbicide activity compared with PVI, especially over viruses [10]. Furthermore, it is not sporicidal and not able to act on biofilms. Nevertheless, it is equally valid for infectious prophylaxis in ocular surgery, especially in cases with confirmed PVI allergy [6, 10].

Topical application on periocular skin must not exceed 0.5% considering the risk of accidental exposure to the corneal epithelium which may cause damage to the corneal epithelium. The recommended concentration for conjunctival irrigation of aqueous chlorhexidine is 0.05 acetate and 0.1% gluconate [10]. Alcoholic chlorhexidine must be avoided because it is toxic to corneal epithelium, stroma and endothelium [10]. Aqueous chlorhexidine is well tolerated, offering low epithelial toxicity [10]. A rare resistance to chlorhexidine of some *Staphylococcus* species has been described [11].

The ozonized oil is an alternative antiseptic in liposomal formulation to improve eye tolerance. The mechanism of action is based on oxygenated compounds, lipidic peroxides and oxygen-reactive species able to damage pathogens through direct oxidation as by interaction with macromolecules, destroying them. Results in animal models and in patients where they show the ability to reduce the ocular surface flora before cataract surgery are promising [12, 13].

3. Antibiotics

Antibiotics have been used during the perioperative period as a prophylactic agent in multiple ophthalmic surgeries. Their use is limited because of the development of antiseptic agents and multiple disadvantages. In fact, antibiotics compared with antiseptics have the following limitations:

- Limited spectrum of antimicrobial activity

- Usually, microbiostatics not microbicides
- High risk of resistance
- Limited or absent activity against multi-resistant organisms
- No residual effect
- Low concentration in the eye
- Cytotoxicity
- Potentially high allergenicity

Antibiotics compared with antiseptics can be used not only topically but also systemically. Topical administrated antibiotics have been most commonly used in ophthalmology, but they did not show superiority compared with antiseptics as prophylactic agents [11].

Alternative administering ways such as systemic, subconjunctival or mixed with irrigation infusion fluid did not show advantages in preventing infections after cataract surgery [1]. Nevertheless, intracameral antibiotics are useful in preventing infectious endo-ophthalmitis after cataract surgery [1, 14]. Intracameral antibiotics can be used at relatively high concentrations and with an extremely low chance of developing microbial resistance [3].

3.1 Intracameral antibiotics

The use of intracameral antibiotics at the end of the cataract surgery is the only procedure that has shown efficacy in endophthalmitis prophylaxis. Generally, three antibiotics have been used: cefuroxime, moxifloxacin and vancomycin, each one of them with their particularities (**Table 1**) [2].

3.1.1 Cefuroxime

Cefuroxime was the antibiotic chosen for the study by the European Society of Cataract and Refractive Surgeons (ESCRS) [1] for its spectrum and experience of use. It is a second-generation cephalosporine that has demonstrated its safety at the doses used for intracameral injection. Although penicillin allergy is frequent, the cross-reactions with cefuroxime are rare. A meta-analysis has estimated that in patients with a history of allergy to penicillin, the general index of cross-reactivity with cephalosporin antibiotics is approximately 1% [15]. The risk of cross-reactivity with penicillin exists principally for first- and second-generations which have similar R1 lateral chains. The cefuroxime has not a similar R1 lateral chain and high risk of cross-reactivity with penicillin is practically negligible, although there are documented cases of anaphylaxis after intracameral use [3].

3.1.2 Moxifloxacin

Moxifloxacin is a fourth-generation fluoroquinolone that inhibits the bacterial topoisomerases II and IV. Intracameral moxifloxacin has not been evaluated in

Antibiotic and recommended dose	Spectrum	Resistances	Security
Cefuroxime 1 mg/0.1 mL	Wide spectrum gram-positive and limited to gram-negative	No efficacy against methicillin-resistant *Staphylococcus. aureus*	Secure at recommended dose. Possibility of toxic anterior segment syndrome at wrong concentrations
Moxifloxacin 250 μg/0.05 mL 0500 μg/0.1 ml	Wide spectrum gram-positive and negative. Good activity against atypical germs	No efficacy against methicillin-resistant *Staphylococcus aureus.* Cross-resistance with other quinolones	Use from the eye drops formulation, without approval for intracameral use
Vancomycin 1 mg/0.1 mL	Effective against the majority of gram-positive. Limited activity against gram-negatives	Rare resistance to gram-positive	Pharmaceutical preparation from intravenous solutions

Table 1.
Characteristics of the antibiotics more used in the prophylaxis in cataract surgery.

randomized clinical trials but the evidence in observational studies suggests that it is effective. A study with more than two million cataract surgeries from the same institution in India showed a general reduction in the number of postoperative endophthalmitis from 0.07 to 0.02% with the routine use of moxifloxacin [2].

There are no anaphylaxis cases reported after the intracameral use and the severe hypersensitivity reactions related to the moxifloxacin are probably rare [2].

3.1.3 Vancomycin

Vancomycin is a glycopeptide antibiotic that acts by binding pentapeptides, preventing peptidoglycans polymerization and weakening bacterial cellular walls [2]. The spectrum of action includes gram-positive coccus, the most frequent causal agent in infectious endophthalmitis. It has been used extensively in the past, but it has gradually been replaced by cefuroxime and moxifloxacin. Intracameral vancomycin 1 mg/0.1 ml is enough to achieve the minimal inhibitory concentration for almost all gram-positive coccus [2]. There are some reasons to avoid it: (1) risk of hemorrhagic/obstructive retinal vasculitis with devastating results on VA; (2) vancomycin is the treatment of choice in infectious endophthalmitis and the use as a prophylactic agent may limit its use if necessary; (3) risk of resistance [2, 11].

3.2 Topical antibiotics

There is no evidence that they are useful in preventing postoperative endophthalmitis when used in the preoperative and postoperative periods [1]. There is evidence that the use of topical antibiotics before surgery is not better than the use of PVI alone [4]. Furthermore, there is a higher risk of resistance and global costs are significantly increased [11]. Nevertheless, postoperative topical antibiotics are commonly used all around the world, especially fluoroquinolones, tobramycin and the combination of polymyxin- neomycin- gramicidin [16].

4. Recommendations for infectious prophylaxis in cataract surgery

Infectious endophthalmitis after cataract surgery is uncommon (0.01-0.08%) [1]. Topical PVI in periocular skin and conjunctival sac and intracameral cefuroxime at the end of the surgery have been demonstrated to be effective as prophylactic measures [1].

Preoperative prophylaxis [1]

- PVI (level of evidence 2, clinical recommendation B): PVI 5% for cleaning of the cornea and conjunctival sac; PVI 10% on periocular skin; minimum recommended contact time: 3 minutes; in case of PVI allergy change to aqueous chlorhexidine 0.05% in the conjunctival sac

- Preoperative lid hygiene (level of evidence 3, clinical recommendation C): can be useful in patients with an increased population of *Staphylococcus aureus* (especially patients with rosacea and atopy)

- Preoperative topical antibiotics (level of evidence 3, clinical recommendation C): there is no evidence of endophthalmitis reduction which can result in resistance.

- Operating room, surgeon and patient preparation: standard protocols of sterilization and operating room preparation. It is important to isolate the eyelashes and eyelids with an adhesive cloth

Recent data suggests PVI 0.5–1% may have the same results as PVI 5% in the conjunctival sac avoiding corneal toxicity and being commercially available also in combination with hyaluronic acid [1]. Nevertheless, these concentrations must be used carefully and according to posology [4].

Intraoperative prophylaxis

- Intracameral antibiotic (level of evidence 1b; clinical recommendation A): cefuroxime (1 mg/0.1 ml) is the preferred antibiotic because: is active against bacteria most commonly involved in endophthalmitis; there is evidence of effectiveness in a European multicentric study; cross-reaction with penicillin is uncommon; availability of a commercial single dose formulation. In allergic patients' moxifloxacin (250-500 µg/0.1 ml) can be used.

In addition to intracameral antibiotics, it is important to confirm that the surgical wound is well sealed at the end of the surgery. In fact, periocular flora is responsible for the vast majority of postsurgical endophthalmitis [17] and if there is any doubt about wound tightness a surgical suture is recommended [18].

Postoperative prophylaxis

Postoperative topical antibiotics are extensively used but their use combined with intracameral antibiotics does not improve results [1, 16]. When used, it is important to avoid a descending treatment regimen because of the risk of improving resistance [11, 18].

5. Conclusions

Topical antiseptics such as PVI have several advantages over antibiotics as prophylactic agents for infectious endophthalmitis after cataract surgery. PVI 5% in the conjunctival sac and PVI 10% on periocular skin for 3 minutes is recommended prior to any cataract surgery to reduce the risk of postoperative endophthalmitis. In patients with an allergy to PVI, chlorhexidine 0.02-0.1% in the conjunctival sac can be used. Intracameral cefuroxime at the end of the surgery is effective as a prophylactic measure, although in allergic patients intracameral moxifloxacin may be used. On the contrary, there is no evidence that postoperative topical antibiotics are useful.

Author details

Sara Crespo Millas[1], Salvatore Di Lauro[1,2*] and David Galarreta Mira[1,2]

1 Hospital Clinico Univeristario de Valladolid, Valladolid, Spain

2 Instituto Oftalmologico Recoletas, Valladolid, Spain

*Address all correspondence to: sadilauro@live.it

References

[1] Barry P, Cordovés L, Gardner S. ESCRS Guidelines for Prevention and Treatment of Endophthalmitis Following Cataract Surgery. Ireland: European Society of Cataract and Refractive Surgeons; 2013

[2] Grzybowski A, Brona P, Zeman L, Stewart MW. Commonly used intracameral antibiotics for endophthalmitis prophylaxis: A literature review. Survey of Ophthalmology. 2021;**66**(1):98-108. Epub 2020/04/29

[3] Haripriya A, Baam ZR, Chang DF. Endophthalmitis prophylaxis for cataract surgery. Asia-Pacific Journal of Ophthalmology (Philadelphia, Pa). 2017;**6**(4):324-329. Epub 2017/08/07

[4] Matsuura K, Miyazaki D, Sasaki SI, Inoue Y, Sasaki Y, Shimizu Y. Effectiveness of intraoperative iodine in cataract surgery: Cleanliness of the surgical field without preoperative topical antibiotics. Japanese Journal of Ophthalmology. 2020;**64**(1):37-44. Epub 2019/11/30

[5] Koerner JC, George MJ, Meyer DR, Rosco MG, Habib MM. Povidone-iodine concentration and dosing in cataract surgery. Survey of Ophthalmology. 2018;**63**(6):862-868. Epub 2018/05/21

[6] Grzybowski A, Kanclerz P, Myers WG. The use of povidone-iodine in ophthalmology. Current Opinion in Ophthalmology. 2018;**29**(1):19-32. Epub 2017/10/07

[7] Modjtahedi BS, van Zyl T, Pandya HK, Leonard RE 2nd, Eliott D. Endophthalmitis after Intravitreal injections in patients with self-reported iodine allergy. American Journal of Ophthalmology. 2016;**170**:68-74. Epub 2016/07/28

[8] Avery RL, Bakri SJ, Blumenkranz MS, Brucker AJ, Cunningham ET Jr, DJ DA, et al. Intravitreal injection technique and monitoring: Updated guidelines of an expert panel. Retina (Philadelphia, Pa). 2014;**34**(Suppl 12):S1-S18. Epub 2014/12/10

[9] Wulf NR, Schmitz J, Choi A, Kapusnik-Uner J. Iodine allergy: Common misperceptions. American Journal of Health-system Pharmacy: AJHP: Official Journal of the American Society of Health-System Pharmacists. 2021;**78**(9):781-793. Epub 2021/02/07

[10] Ali FS, Jenkins TL, Boparai RS, Obeid A, Ryan ME, Wibblesman TD, et al. Aqueous chlorhexidine compared with povidone-iodine as ocular antisepsis before Intravitreal injection: A randomized clinical trial. Ophthalmology Retina. 2021;**5**(8):788-796. Epub 2020/11/23

[11] Grzybowski A, Brona P, Kim SJ. Microbial flora and resistance in ophthalmology: A review. Graefe's Archive for Clinical and Experimental Ophthalmology = Albrecht von Graefes Archiv fur klinische und experimentelle Ophthalmologie. 2017;**255**(5):851-862. Epub 2017/02/24

[12] Marchegiani A, Magagnini M, Cerquetella M, Troiano P, Franchini I, Franchini A, et al. Preoperative topical liposomal ozone dispersion to reduce bacterial colonization in conjunctival sac and periocular skin: Preliminary study in dogs. Experimental Eye Research. 2019;**189**:107848. Epub 2019/10/22

[13] Pérez-Santonja JJ, Güell JL, Gris O, Vázquez Dorrego XM, Pellicer E, Benítez-Del-Castillo JM. Liposomal Ozonated oil in ocular infections: A review of preclinical and clinical

studies, focusing on its antiseptic and regenerative properties. Clinical Ophthalmology (Auckland, NZ). 2022;**16**:1953-1962. Epub 2022/06/22

[14] Linertová R, Abreu-González R, García-Pérez L, Alonso-Plasencia M, Cordovés-Dorta LM, Abreu-Reyes JA, et al. Intracameral cefuroxime and moxifloxacin used as endophthalmitis prophylaxis after cataract surgery: Systematic review of effectiveness and cost-effectiveness. Clinical Ophthalmology (Auckland, NZ). 2014;**8**:1515-1522. Epub 2014/08/26

[15] Campagna JD, Bond MC, Schabelman E, Hayes BD. The use of cephalosporins in penicillin-allergic patients: A literature review. The Journal of Emergency Medicine. 2012;**42**(5):612-620. Epub 2011/07/12

[16] Vazirani J, Basu S. Role of topical, subconjunctival, intracameral, and irrigative antibiotics in cataract surgery. Current Opinion in Ophthalmology. 2013;**24**(1):60-65. Epub 2012/10/20

[17] Speaker MG, Milch FA, Shah MK, Eisner W, Kreiswirth BN. Role of external bacterial flora in the pathogenesis of acute postoperative endophthalmitis. Ophthalmology. 1991;**98**(5):639-649 . discussion 50. Epub 1991/05/01

[18] Olson RJ, Braga-Mele R, Chen SH, Miller KM, Pineda R 2nd, Tweeten JP, et al. Cataract in the adult eye preferred practice pattern®. Ophthalmology. 2017;**124**(2):P1-P119. Epub 2016/10/18

Chapter 2

Corneal Disease and Its Impact on Cataract Surgery

Brian A. Bird, Albert Y. Cheung and John D. Sheppard

Abstract

The primary focus of this book chapter is to investigate and discuss the impact of corneal disease and how various types of corneal pathology can affect the surgeons preop, intraop and post op management when considering cataract surgery for a patient. Cataract surgery is known to exacerbate ocular surface diseases like dry eye, HSV, inflammatory conditions like ocular cicatricial pemphigoid, SJS, peripheral ulcerative keratitis, Moorens ulcer and endothelial disease like Fuch's dystrophy secondary to intraoperative endothelial cell loss. Preoperative treatment including optimization of the corneal surface, antiviral prophylaxis in HSV keratitis, quiescence of inflammation and preoperative diagnostic evaluation of endothelial cell counts may all play a role in postoperative outcomes. Corneal disease may also impact intraoperative considerations in cataract extraction to include the use of scleral tunnels or even Extracapsular Cataract extraction techniques, for example, in patients with Mooren's ulcer to decrease corneal melt. More commonly corneal disease consequently provides a poor view for the surgeon and unfavorable post op visual acuity for the patient. Consideration of staged keratoplasty and cataract surgery vs. combined "triple procedure" have both been shown as reasonable treatment options. Postoperative considerations include management of endothelial cell loss during surgery and minimizing postoperative eye drops and medicomentosa.

Keywords: cornea, cataract surgery, dry eye, triple procedure, keratoplasty, corneal scar

1. Introduction

Cataracts are the world's leading cause of blindness in patients age 50 and older [1], and consequently, cataract surgery is a common ophthalmological procedure. This chapter focuses on the considerations regarding coexisting corneal disease and how various corneal diseases affect cataract surgery preoperatively, intraoperatively, and postoperatively.

2. Ocular surface disease

2.1 Dry eye disease (DED)

Dry eye is a multifactorial disease of the ocular surface characterized by a loss of homoeostasis of the tear film, and a vicious cycle of inflammation on the ocular surface. Generally, DED is classified as aqueous deficient (e.g., secondary to Sjogrens syndrome) or evaporative (e.g., secondary to Meibomian gland dysfunction). This classification can help direct the ophthalmologists when developing an approach to treatment. DED is a critical entity to manage properly perioperatively as it is ubiquitous among cataract patients, can be worsened by surgical disruption of the tear film and postoperative drops, and can have a profound effect on postoperative visual acuity with consequences of patient satisfaction. Prevalence rates are estimated to range from 5 to 50% and as high as 75% in adults over 40 [2, 3]. Patient symptoms include burning, itching, epiphora, and decreased visual acuity. A basic understanding of the anatomy and physiology that contributes to a healthy ocular surface is helpful to understand when tailoring a treatment plan. The Lacrimal Functional Unit (LFU) is a term used to include the lacrimal glands, ocular surface, eyelids and the motor and sensory nerves that connect and regulate these structures. A healthy LFU is responsible for maintaining a healthy tear film, and for maintaining a healthy transparent corneal surface to project a crisp image onto the retina. The eyelids contribute by protecting the ocular surface; blinking which distributes the tear film across the eye and stimulates the lacrimal gland to pump tears out onto the surface of the eye; and producing secretions that contribute to the tear film. Lagophthalmos can be seen secondary to facial nerve palsies from strokes and diseases like Bell's Palsy, HSV, VZV, and Lyme disease. The secretions (e.g., meibum) from the eyelid primarily help in reducing evaporative loss of tears [4]. Dysregulation of any of these components can contribute to DED.

2.2 Preoperative evaluation

In regards to dryness, the preoperative examination is a crucial step in identifying eyes that need ocular surface optimization prior to cataract surgery. Dryness can be exacerbated by cataract surgery, so treatment preoperatively can decrease the chance of a severely decompensated ocular surface postoperatively. Dryness can have a significant effect in altering the tear film and cornea with consequential effects on preoperative biometry measurements, namely the inaccuracy and variability of keratometry readings. For example, Epitropolous et al. looked at a cohort of 100 hyperosmolar (a point-of-care marker for dryness) and 50 normal eyes and found that the hyperosmolar group had a statistically significant higher variability of keratometry readings as compared to the normal group. The hyperosmolar group had a higher percentage with 1D or greater difference in measured astigmatism as well as a higher percentage of eyes with an IOL power difference of more than 0.5D [5]. **Figures 1** and **2** show an example of how preoperative treatment of dryness can not only improve the ocular surface but also lead to more accurate measurements and IOL selection.

Slit lamp examination can be used to visualize underlying causes of DED to help direct the surgeon's treatment approach. Meibomian gland dysfunction (MGD), demodex collarettes, punctal stenosis, entropion, ectropion, lagophthalmos, and

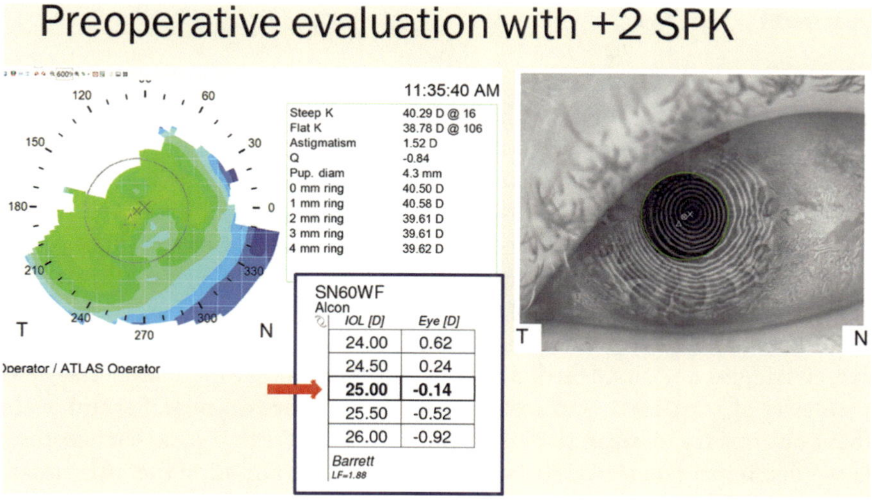

Figure 1.
Preoperative keratometry readings and intraocular lens selection in a patient with 2+ SPK. Note the irregular topography and mires on right and left images, respectively.

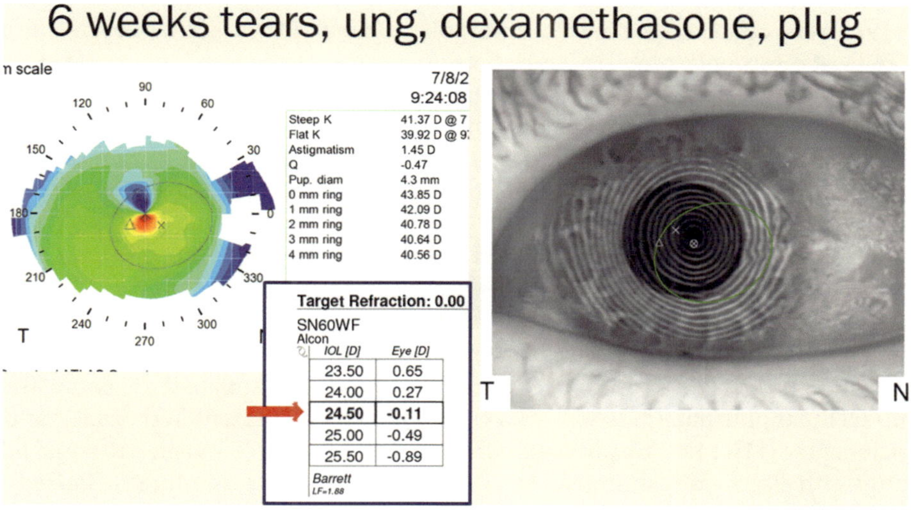

Figure 2.
For the same eye in **Figure 1***, repeat measurements after 6 weeks of treatment with artificial tears, ointment, preservative free dexamethasone twice daily, and punctal plugs demonstrate improved topography and mires as well as a change in the IOL selection.*

floppy eyelids can be identified and targeted to optimize the ocular surface preoperatively. Fluorescein and vital dye stains can be used to visualize superficial punctate keratitis (SPK). In addition to the slit lamp exam, several clinical and diagnostic tests are used for the diagnosis and the management of DED. A tear break-up time of less than 10 seconds is considered abnormal and supports an evaporative component of dry eye disease commonly seen in MGD. Interferometry and infrared meibography may also help with diagnosis and follow-up. The Schirmer 1 and 2 tests investigate tear production. Tear osmolarity, IgE, and MMP 9 are all point-of-care tests that analyze the composition of the tears themselves.

2.3 Treatment

Given the many available treatment options for DED, a tailored approach is best for these patients when optimizing the ocular surface in preparation for cataract surgery. For cases of mild dryness or an unstable tear film, a relatively quick regimen of aggressive preservative free lubrication [6] (e.g., tears, ointment) and corticosteroids (often only short-term, e.g. preservative free dexamethasone), with punctal occlusion if necessary, may be all the eye needs for better preoperative testing. It is good to maintain the dry eye therapy perioperatively as cataract surgery and the required postoperative drops can disrupt the tear film and cause additional dryness.

One of the challenges of managing DED is that it stimulates an inflammatory cascade which triggers a positive feedback loop of inflammatory mediators that increase the osmolarity of tears further exacerbating ocular surface dryness. Several of the treatment options try to break the inflammatory cycle. Weak topical corticosteroids can have a fast impact on the ocular surface. Treatments targeting the inflammatory component of DED may be necessary to break the cycle of inflammation in moderate to severe disease. Cyclosporine A is available in three formulations Restasis, Cequa, and now a generic form is available. In large phase 3 trials, both Restasis and Cequa have proven effective in increasing tear production as measured by Schirmer testing [7, 8], and subsequent studies have shown that cyclosporine may also increase goblet cells [9]. In the context of cataract surgery, one study of 28 eyes showed cyclosporine 0.05% used one month preop to 2 months post op improved visual quality after multifocal IOL implantation [10]. Other treatments that target the inflammatory component of dry eye disease include topical corticosteroid drops (Eyesuvis) and lifitegrast ophthalmic solution (Xiidra), an LFA-1 antagonist thereby inhibiting LFA-1 binding to overexpressed ICAM-1. Autologous serum tears have also been used to treat severe dry eyes.

To address blepharitis and meibomian gland dysfunction, eyelid hygiene including warm compresses and lid sprays or wipes work to increase meibomian gland secretions and remove debris. Oral low-dose doxycycline may also be used to obtain a quick response to treating the lids through its anti-inflammatory and lipid layer stabilization properties. Azithromycin has been found to stimulate the accumulation of intracellular phospholipids and lysozymes which are important in the maturation of meibocytes [11]. Microblepharoexfoliation treatment (e.g. Blephex), thermal lid therapy with gland expression (e.g. Lipiflow, TearCare, iLux), and Intense Pulsed Light (IPL) therapies are procedures that are designed to increase meibomian gland secretions onto the ocular surface; several studies have shown them to be effective treatment options as well [12–16]. These can potentially help combat lid disease quickly prior to cataract surgery. Moisture chamber goggles, sutured tarsorrhaphies and lid weights can all be utilized to prevent evaporative tear loss from the eye. When appropriate, addressing the lid malposition (e.g., ectropion/entropion) may be necessary to help the ocular surface. If the underlying cause of DED is Neurotrophic Keratitis, cenegermin (Oxervate) is a FDA approved drug that works directly upon corneal epithelial cells and corneal nociceptors as recombinant nerve growth factor [17, 18].

2.4 Intraoperative considerations

As illustrated above, dry eye disease can cause decreased visual acuity for the patient and by the same mechanism can cause decreased clarity through the irregular cornea during cataract surgery. To optimize the surgeons view, a dispersive ophthalmic viscosurgical device can be applied to the cornea to decrease dryness during surgery. If the ocular surface dryness is secondary to neurotrophic keratitis the surgeon should minimize additional nerve damage by avoiding the use of limbal relaxing incisions and multiple paracentesis wounds (e.g., using Malyugin ring instead of iris hooks) when possible. Similarly, limbal relaxing incisions should be avoided. At the end of the case, the surgeon may consider the addition of a bandage contact lens or in more severe cases of ocular surface or tarsorrhaphy may be considered. Dropless cataract surgery (e.g., transzonular or intravitreal injectables, resorbable dexamethasone punctal plugs) may be used to minimize medicamentosa along with avoiding/decreasing postoperative topical NSAIDs.

3. Ocular inflammatory diseases

Severe ocular surface inflammatory conditions such as Peripheral Ulcerative Keratitis (PUK), graft vs. host disease (GVHD), Stevens Johnson Syndrome (SJS), mucous membrane pemphigoid (MMP), and Mooren's Ulcer may need additional preop/postop care and surgical planning due to disease sequelae (e.g. corneal thinning and scarring, conjunctival and limbal stem cell deficiency) and the potential risk of reactivation of disease (e.g. corneal thinning).

3.1 Preoperative evaluation

Obtaining relevant past medical history can be important, especially with attention to rheumatological conditions such as rheumatoid arthritis, spondyloarthritides, and other inflammatory arthritides/systemic disorders. Slit Lamp examination can reveal evidence of current and prior ocular surface inflammation including corneal scarring/thinning, corneal neovascularization, limbal stem cell failure, symblepharon formation, dry eye, and associated uveitis. Conjunctival injection can be a good surrogate marker of current inflammation level or control. Evaluating for signs of dry eye (as above) and appropriate preoperative management are critical for success postoperatively. If there is conjunctival inflammation or associated uveitis, it is important to have the eye quiet for at least 3 months prior to surgical intervention. If there is significant thinning, a pachymap can be useful to determine the best incision placement. Once the diagnosis has been made, the goal is to control inflammation before cataract surgery; otherwise, the surgery may exacerbate inflammation and can lead to worse outcomes. Potentially, control of these diseases requires systemic immunosuppression with collaboration with a rheumatologist, and patient specific surgical planning is critical (**Figure 3**) [19–22].

3.2 Intraoperative considerations

Having a surgical plan can be quite helpful in these eyes. Base incisions locations from a pachymap or preoperative slit lamp examination to avoid areas of vascularization and thinning. It may be necessary to consider a scleral tunnel if there is a history of corneal melts or thin limbal inadequate areas to make an incision. A study of 15 eyes with MMP showed that cataract surgery could be done successfully on these eyes but recommended the use of small corneal incisions to reduce the risk of conjunctival inflammation [19]. In contrast, patients with a Mooren's ulcer may require scleral

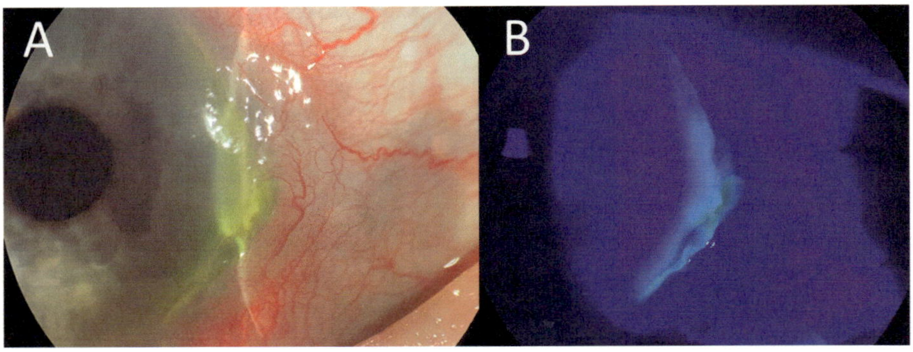

Figure 3.
Slit lamp photograph of peripheral ulcerative keratitis in a patient with rheumatoid arthritis with slit beam highlighting the thinned area (A) and fluorescein highlighting the epithelial defect (B).

tunnel wounds or even extracapsular cataract extraction to minimize risk of triggering corneal melt [22]. Trypan blue is often useful when there is corneal scarring/opacity to optimize capsulorrhexis creation when visualization is not ideal. A suture may be necessary to help seal incisions when there is adjacent scarring or thinning. A bandage contact lens can be placed at the end of the case to protect the cornea and facilitate rehabilitation of the ocular surface. A subconjunctival or subtenons injection of corticosteroid can be helpful in controlling postoperative inflammation.

3.3 Postoperative management

These eyes require closer follow-up postoperatively as they are at higher risk for ocular surface decompensation, keratolysis, and chronic/recurrent uveitis. When dryness appears to worsen, consider a decrease in particular drops such as NSAIDS to avoid drop toxicity. NSAIDS may even need to be avoided in patients with an increased risk of keratolysis based on past ocular (history of prior melts) and medical history (e.g. GVHD, rheumatoid arthritis). Aggressive DED management can help prevent worsening disease with sequelae such as erosions and melting. Depending on the degree of irregular astigmatism, a rigid gas permeable lens may be needed for best visual acuity after cataract surgery and should be discussed with the patient preoperatively.

4. Pterygia

A pterygium occurs from elastotic degeneration and leads to fibrovascular growth of the limbal/interpalpebral conjunctiva onto the cornea. Despite its benign nature, pterygia can be progressive with further growth toward the visual axis and increased irregular astigmatism.

4.1 Preoperative evaluation

Slit lamp examination is important to determine how far the pterygium extends over the cornea. Other aspects such as injection, elevation, calcifications, underlying fibrosis/scarring, associated thinning, and healthy conjunctiva elsewhere can be helpful for preoperative planning and to establish medical necessity for excision. Topography can help demonstrate the magnitude of irregular astigmatism (often flattening) and how close to the paracentral/midperipheral cornea this encroaches. Placido disk corneal topography can be particularly useful as one can view the distortion of mires from the pterygium.

There are different approaches to the timing of pterygium excision in the setting of planning cataract surgery. If the pterygium is not affecting the midperipheral cornea or more central (and topography is not greatly affected), cataract surgery may be considered without any pterygium surgery. The pterygium is typically less than 2–3 mm encroachment onto the cornea in this setting. Kim et al. noted that pterygia <2.0 mm rarely induce postoperative changes after removal [23]. The patient should be aware that the pterygium may need to addressed in the future if best correctable vision is not satisfactory and glasses will likely be necessary for best vision. If visually significant or impacting cataract surgery corneal measurements, pterygium surgery can be performed prior to cataract surgery or simultaneously. If prior to cataract surgery, there should be approximately 3 months between surgeries to allow for stabilization and repeat measurements. This strategy likely allows for the best chance of achieving the desired post-refractive goal following cataract surgery. If the surgeries are performed simultaneously, this has the benefit of only one surgery for patients, but there is a decreased chance of hitting a post-refractive target. Steepening of the cornea can occur resulting in myopia [24], so IOL power selection should take this into account. Studies have noted that the longer or greater the pterygium size, the greater the change in keratometry readings [23, 25, 26]. Toric correction should only be considered when there is regular astigmatism after pterygium removal, and it should be avoided in irregular corneas and inconsistent corneal readings. Multifocal IOLs are often a poor choice when there is irregular astigmatism and higher levels of higher order aberrations. If there is associated fibrosis especially centrally or paracentrally, the patient should understand that a hard lens may be necessary postoperatively to achieve the best vision (**Figure 4**).

4.2 Intraoperative considerations

During cataract surgery, trypan blue may help with visualization if there is central or paracentral scarring. If a temporal small pterygium is present and the plan is to leave it be, the main incision should be positioned elsewhere.

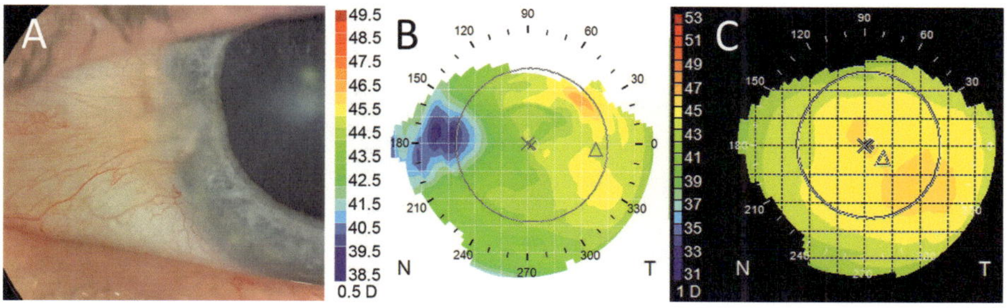

Figure 4.
Slit lamp photograph of a nasal pterygium. Preoperative topography demonstrates nasal flattening with 1.56 D of astigmatism. Following excision with autograft, postoperative topography demonstrates a more regular surface with 0.39 D of astigmatism.

4.3 Postoperative management

While recurrence rates are low (<10%) following conventional pterygium surgery with an autograft, there typically is no deviation from standard cataract surgery in regards to postoperative management. One should continue to monitor pterygium recurrence.

5. Corneal opacification

Corneal scarring, Salzmann nodules, dystrophies (e.g. epithelial basement membrane dystrophy [EBMD]), and band keratopathy can present unique challenges in preoperative measurements, significantly compromise the view of the surgeon during cataract surgery, and may even require staged or simultaneous keratoplasty along with cataract extraction.

5.1 Preoperative evaluation

Preoperative evaluation of corneal opacities include slit lamp examination, assessment of BCVA using the Snellen chart, and ultrasound B-scan if view of the fundus is obscured. The broad slit beam can often highlight the extent of the scarring and improve visualization of EBMD and fibrosis associated with nodules. Fluorescein can highlight the pathology, especially when there is negative staining of areas that are not seen with broad beam lighting. When these corneal changes are seen in the central 5–6 mm, they are more likely to be visually significant or alter preoperative topography measurements. Topography can help demonstrate how much irregular astigmatism is present and how close to the central/paracentral cornea these conditions are affecting. Placido disk corneal topography can be particularly useful as one can view the distortion of mires from the involved pathology. When the view of the cataract is obstructed by the corneal opacity, additional diagnostic testing can include anterior segment optical coherence tomography (ASOCT) which can allow the surgeon to assess the depth of corneal scars, and it can also be used to provide information regarding anterior chamber depth and characteristics of the cataract. A recent literature assessment demonstrated that ASOCT can be used to reveal structural details of the anterior capsule, objective measurements about the cataract itself including white and hypermature cataracts and the stability of the posterior capsule [27]. Another study compared anterior segment OCT to UBM in identifying posterior capsule rupture in traumatic cataracts. They discovered that ASOCT was superior to UBM in terms of its sensitivity, specificity, and positive and negative predictive values [28]. Corneal densitometry can be analyzed by a rotating Scheimpflug camera (Pentacam AXL; Oculus, Wetzlar, Germany). This modality can demonstrate the opaque area of the cornea and provide an objective score from 0 to 100 (most transparent to most opaque respectively).

5.2 Treatment

Superficial keratectomy (SK) is a procedure in which the corneal epithelium is removed and can be utilized if the corneal disease/damage is superficial to Bowman's membrane. EBMD, Salzmann Nodules and band keratopathy are easily addressed with a keratectomy (and EDTA for band keratopathy) when the pathology is obstructing the central 5–6 mm (**Figure 5**).

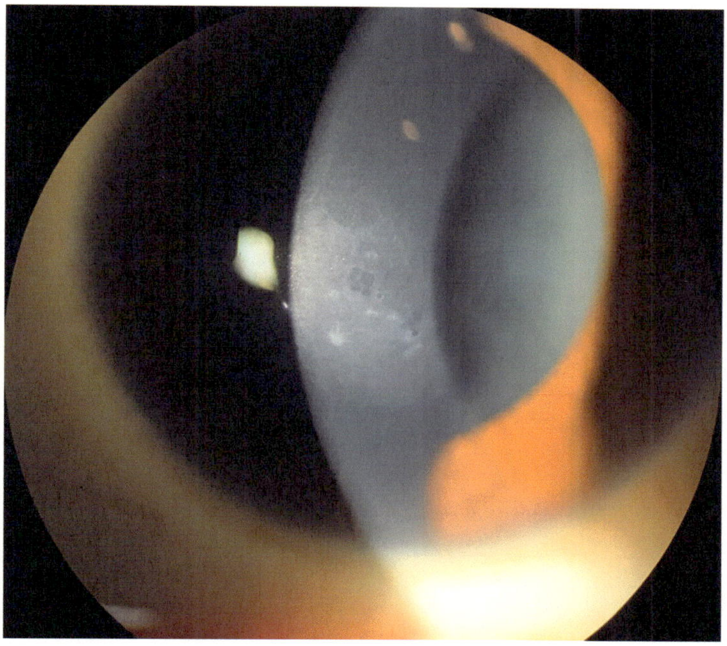

Figure 5.
Slit lamp photograph of epithelial basement membrane dystrophy. This was treated with a superficial keratectomy prior to cataract surgery.

Multiple studies have demonstrated that SK is a safe and effective treatment to improve visual acuity, reduce corneal astigmatism, and optimize biometry readings [29]. A study at Duke specifically looked at the biometry readings of patients with EBMD and Salzmann nodular degeneration pre and post SK or PTK which showed that 21 out of 26 eyes treated for EBMD had a change in predicted IOL power and 16 of 24 eyes had a change in the recommended IOL toricity with a mean cylinder power change of 1.2 diopters. About 11 of 13 eyes with Salzmann Nodular degeneration had a change in predicated IOL power and 10 of the 11 toric eligible eyes had a change in the recommended IOL toricity with a mean cylinder power change of 1.5 diopters (**Figures 6** and 7) [30].

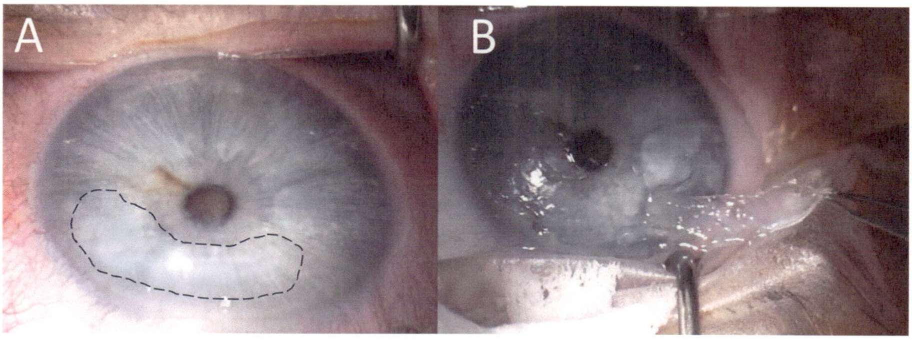

Figure 6.
Intraoperative still photograph demonstrating a superior Salzmann nodule (dotted outline, a). This is peeled off during a superficial keratectomy (B).

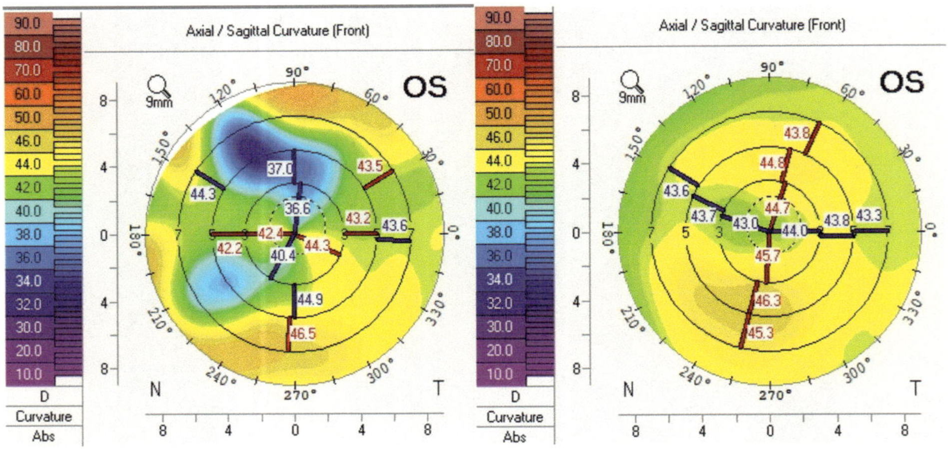

Figure 7.
Topography of an eye with a Salzmann nodule treated with a superficial keratectomy: Preoperative, left (note flattening superiorly) and postoperative, right.

When the corneal opacity is restricted to the anterior 100 uM of the cornea, phototherapeutic keratectomy (PTK) using the 193 nm excimer laser can be considered prior to cataract surgery. The primary indications for PTK include anterior corneal dystrophies, such as lattice, granular, and Reis-Bückler's dystrophy [31]. Corneal degenerations such as Salzmann's nodular degeneration and climatic droplet keratopathy, also can be successfully treated with PTK [32]. Some of the complications associated with PTK include induced myopia, hyperopia, irregular astigmatism, haze, recurrence, and corneal thinning [31, 32]. As such subsequent cataract surgery should be delayed at least 6–12 weeks after PTK, once stabilization of the cornea has been established. A new topical medication losartan (used off-label 0.8 mg/mL six times per day) may help with treatment of certain types of corneal fibrosis/scarring in preparation for surgery (**Figure 8**) [33].

5.3 Intraoperative considerations

Often, the involved pathology is addressed with a keratectomy. In the setting of corneal opacity, trypan blue is safe and has been widely used for better visualization of the anterior capsule [34]. Pupillary enlargement is a technique that can be used

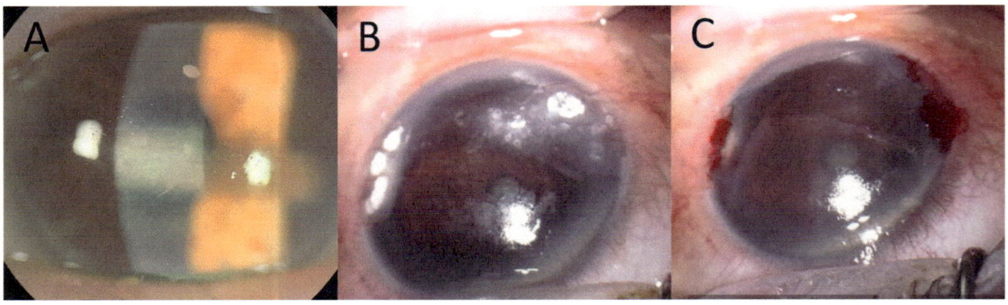

Figure 8.
Slit lamp photograph of band keratopathy (A). Intraoperative still photograph demonstrating another patient with band keratopathy. (B) Demonstrates the preoperative appearance and (C) demonstrates appearance following removal with superficial keratectomy and EDTA application.

to create an optical window via sphincterotomy or an optical iridectomy when the corneal opacity blocks the central visual axis as an alternative to a corneal transplant procedure [35]. Endoillumination is a technique whereby an endoillumination probe is inserted through a corneal paracentesis (or alternatively a transconjunctival chandelier illumination system) to improve visualization during cataract surgery (**Figure 9**) [36, 37].

If the corneal opacification is inhibiting a patients best corrected visual acuity or the surgeons view to safely perform cataract surgery, a keratoplasty may be necessary. Depending on the depth of the corneal opacification, surgical options include a combined surgery referred to as a Triple Procedure, that is, Penetrating Keratoplasty (PKP) or Deep Anterior Lamellar Keratoplasty (DALK) with cataract extraction and IOL implantation) vs. a staged procedure where the keratoplasty is performed first and the cataract surgery is done at a later time (**Figure 10**).

Combined surgery should be considered in patients with health problems that place patients at high risk for undergoing multiple surgeries under anesthesia or for patients whose health/life situation necessitates more rapid visual recovery [38, 39]. In a combined surgery, cataract extraction can be performed via phacoemulsification or via the open sky technique with extracapsular cataract extraction. The main disadvantages in a combined surgery using the open sky technique is that the eye is exposed to the outside environment for a longer time thereby increasing the patient's risk for endophthalmitis, and possible suprachoroidal/expulsive hemorrhage due to acute hypotony. Additionally, patients' postoperative refractive errors are generally higher due to inaccuracy of IOL formulas when the measurements are estimated as well as postoperative changes in keratometric values, AC depth, and axial length [38–42]. Staged surgery is generally more controlled as compared to open sky because it is performed in a closed system [41–43]. Additionally, a staged surgery is more likely to provide the patient with better postoperative vision because it allows for more accurate IOL power calculation due to more accurate preoperative diagnostic testing. As the cornea is allowed to stabilize and astigmatism minimized with suture removal, surgical adjustments such as placement of the main wound at the steep axis of the cornea and placement of arcuate keratotomy can be performed during cataract surgery. Although potentially controversial, toric IOLs can be considered in certain situations; however, they are often avoided with PK and DALK as a future graft replacement would leave a toric IOL with a mismatched cornea. This may not be as significant a factor with the ability to place an endothelial keratoplasty under a PK/

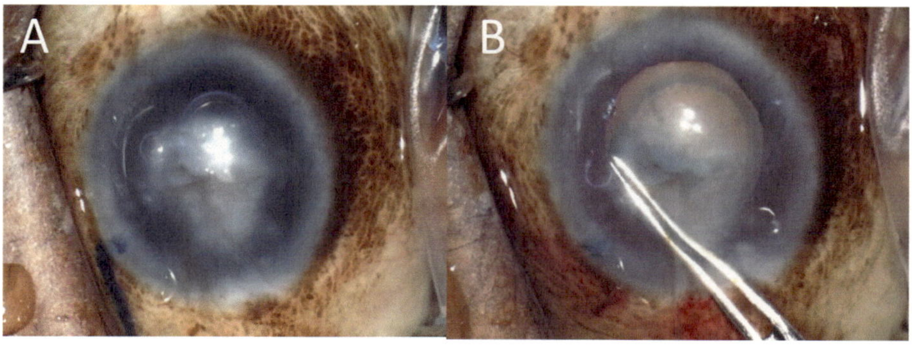

Figure 9.
Intraoperative still photograph demonstrating use of trypan due to poor visualization from corneal scarring/opacity (A) and how this improved ability to perform capsulorrhexis (B).

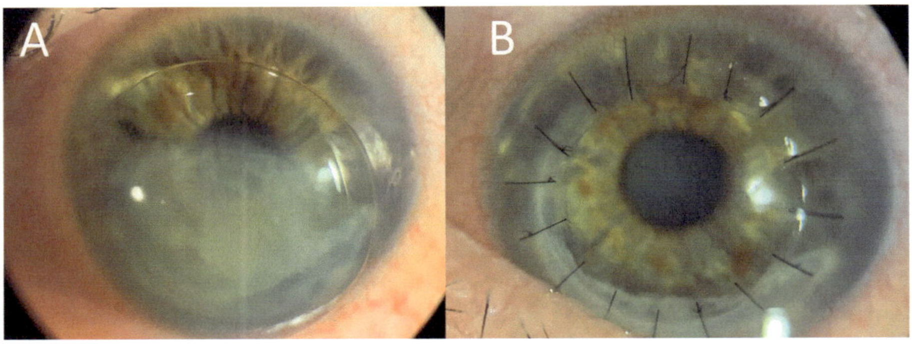

Figure 10.
Slit lamp photograph of dense large scar with overlying rigid gas permeable lens (A). After worsening cataract, it was determined that a deep anterior lamellar keratoplasty would best allow for cataract extraction (B).

DALK. The disadvantages of a staged procedure include endothelial cell loss, the risks of undergoing anesthesia a second time, and the large delay in visual improvement due to the requisite time after keratoplasty for stabilization of keratometric values and suture removal which may take up to 6–12 months [37–39]. When cataract surgery is performed staged under a keratoplasty, trypan blue may be necessary if visualization is poor. A scleral tunnel may be necessary to avoid crossing the graft-host-junction with the main incision. Using extra OVD is prudent to minimize endothelial damage as there is faster endothelial cell attrition for a keratoplasty compared to a native cornea. Sutures are often needed as wounds may gape and leak due to the inherent contraction from the keratoplasty.

5.4 Post operative management

The etiology of the corneal opacification must be taken into consideration in the post operative period as it may help guide the surgeons post operative management. If the corneal scar was originally from HSV/VZV, it is important to place patient on prophylactic oral antiviral due to the increased risk of recurrence of epithelial or stromal disease following intraocular surgery. Close monitoring is especially important postoperatively in patients with corneal disease as patients can have recurrence of corneal pathology and repeat opacification of the cornea. If the visual acuity is not satisfactory following cataract ± corneal surgery an RGP lens may be utilized to minimize the decrease in visual acuity secondary to irregular astigmatism often seen in these patients.

6. Endothelial disease

Due to the potential collateral damage to endothelial cells during cataract surgery, careful consideration and patient specific planning is necessary in the setting of coexisting corneal endothelial disease. While low endothelial cell density can be seen in patients with a history of intraocular inflammation, prior corneal transplant, prior glaucoma filtering surgery, or trauma, it is most commonly encountered in patients with a history of Fuch's corneal dystrophy [44]. Once a cataract becomes visually significant, earlier extraction may be beneficial to minimize damage to endothelial cells, especially if a simultaneous corneal procedure is being avoided.

6.1 Preoperative evaluation

Slit lamp examination of the cataract maturity is important as denser cataracts predictably require more ultrasonic energy and lead to more endothelial cell loss. The status of the cornea should be evaluated at slit lamp specifically looking for guttata, edema, and fibrosis from longstanding stromal edema which can all diminish a patient's best corrected vision and may also impair the surgeons view into the anterior chamber during cataract surgery. Any preoperative clinical signs of corneal edema warrant consideration of addressing the endothelial function at the time of cataract surgery (**Figure 11**).

While pachymetry and specular microscopy classically were used to determine risk of corneal decompensation following cataract surgery, these may be poor measures of prognosis. Unless there was a baseline pachymetry taken years ago, pachymetry is not often useful as it may not correlate well with edema. Tomography may be a more useful tool in evaluating early Fuchs prior to cataract surgery. Sun et al. created tomography criteria that can be helpful to evaluate Fuchs eyes to determine subclinical edema. These include loss of parallel isopachs, displacement of the thinnest point of the cornea, and focal posterior corneal surface depression [45]. Another study from this group also evaluated the risk for progression of Fuchs and/or needing surgical intervention following uncomplicated cataract surgery using the same criteria. Risk was 0% when no criteria/patterns were present, 50% when any 1 or 2 of the criteria/patterns were present, and 75% when all 3 were present [46]. Given the possibility for needing a surgical intervention, it can be prudent to aim myopic for the post-refractive goal as endothelial keratoplasty will often cause a hyperopic shift. To account for this, aiming for −0.50 to −0.75, −1.00, and − 1.00 to 1.25 sphere for DMEK, nano-thin DSEK, and ultrathin DSEK, respectively. Avoid placing a hydrophilic intraocular lens given the possibility of calcification with these following the gas/air with an endothelial keratoplasty (**Figure 12**).

6.2 Intraoperative considerations

Factors that increase the risk of endothelial cell loss during cataract surgery include longer phacoemulsification time such as that required with denser cataracts and shorter axial length [47]. Care should be taken to refill the anterior chamber to

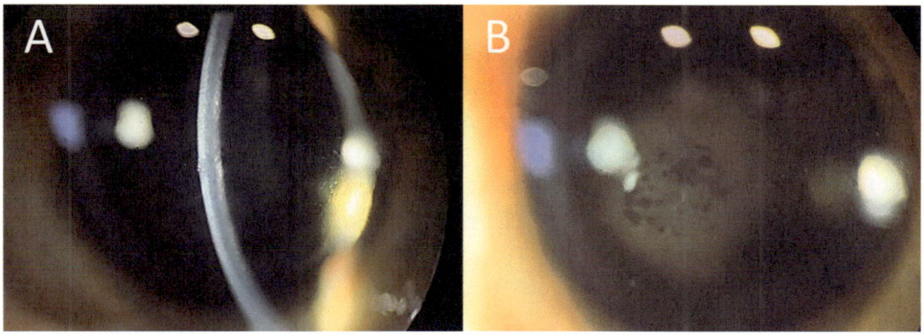

Figure 11.
Slit lamp photograph with slit beam (A) demonstrating guttata and corneal edema with anterior haze and microcystic edema in an eye with Fuchs corneal dystrophy. This is highlighted with sclerotic scatter lighting technique to demonstrate the microcystic edema and bullae (B).

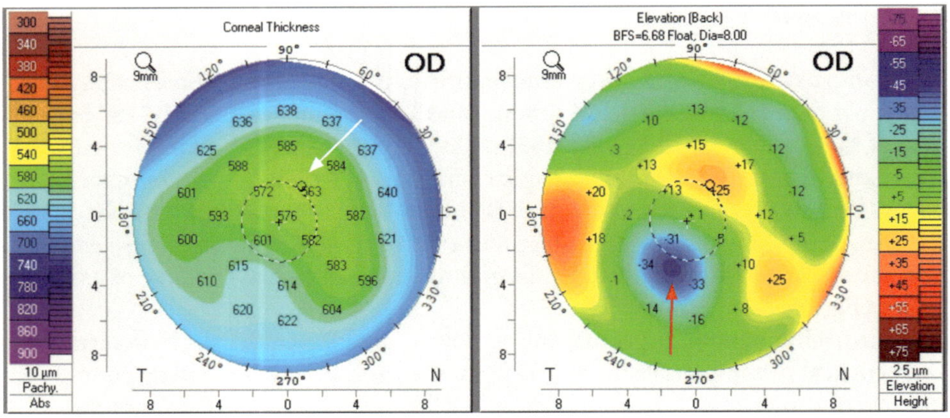

Figure 12.
Preoperative tomography in an eye with Fuchs demonstrates loss of parallel oval/circular isopachs, displacement of the thinnest point of the cornea (white arrow), and focal posterior corneal surface depression (red arrow).

coat the endothelium with dispersive viscoelastic between cataract quadrants/segments in these situations. Systemic illnesses may also increase the risk of endothelial cell loss during cataract surgery. One study investigated endothelial cell loss in diabetic patients undergoing cataract surgery as compared to non-diabetics and showed a significant increase in endothelial cell loss 3 months postoperatively in the diabetic study group [48]. Surgical treatment options for patients with cataract and coexisting endothelial disease include cataract surgery alone or combined surgeries (with either a simultaneous triple procedure or staged). Combined options include DMEK with phacoemulsification and IOL placement, DSAEK with phacoemulsification and IOL placement, DSO with phacoemulsification and IOL placement. Factors that may determine a simultaneous compared to stage procedure include degree of cornea vs. lens pathology, post-refractive goals (may be more accurate with corneal surgery and repeat measurements prior to cataract surgery), and patient preference (1 surgery versus 2 surgeries). Torics may be considered for mild Fuchs with a clear regular corneal cylinder on topography of more than 2 diopters. It may be better to stage toric IOL given the hypotony and anterior chamber shallowing during endothelial keratoplasty (especially DMEK) which could potentially rotate the IOL.

Trypan blue can be useful to see through dense guttata especially in corneal haze or bullae are associated. If edema is severe, one may perform a keratectomy to improve the view. If performing cataract surgery alone, phacoemulsification at iris plane (more posterior) may decrease endothelial damage, while phacoemulsification near the cornea in combined surgery is fine as the endothelium will be replaced and damage to the posterior capsule can be minimized. Additionally, a smaller capsulorrhexis may be better for combined cases to keep the IOL in the capsular bag during anterior chamber shallowing; similarly, using only cohesive viscoelastic in combined cases can allow for less chance of having retained viscoelastic in the graft interface.

6.3 Postoperative management

Postoperatively, patients with Fuchs should be counseled that there may be delayed deturgescence of their corneas following cataract surgery. This may even take several weeks to a couple months, and topical sodium chloride can be helpful. If the edema fails to clear, one can then consider endothelial surgery. In the setting of Fuchs

DOI: http://dx.doi.org/10.5772/intechopen.1002404

post-cataract surgery, it can be prudent to avoid a large YAG treatment to minimize vitreous prolapse into the anterior chamber with future endothelial keratoplasty (especially DMEK).

7. Keratoconus

Keratoconus is a corneal ectatic disease resulting in irregular astigmatism often characterized by inferior steepening of the cornea, irregularities in the corneal stroma and breaks in Bowman's layer. Risk factors for keratoconus include patients' with connective tissue disease, Down syndrome, and patient's with atopic disease or habitual eye rubbing [49]. The onset of keratoconus is generally in adolescence and tends to stabilize by 30–40 years of age [50, 51]. Treatment options include hard contact lenses, intrastromal corneal ring segments, corneal cross linking, and DALK or PKP in later stages of the disease. Patients with keratoconus tend to develop cataracts at a younger age [52] and successful surgical treatment of cataracts in patients with keratoconus requires additional considerations in the preoperative and intraoperative period (**Figure 13**).

7.1 Preoperative evaluation

Most notably in the preoperative period, one of the challenges in keratoconus is obtaining reliable IOL power measurements due to unreliable keratometric values and potentially different anatomy (increased axial length and anterior chamber depth leading to more posterior effective lens position) [53]. As keratoconus is a progressive disease, stability of disease should ideally be demonstrated before cataract surgery should be attempted. The Global Consensus on Keratoconus and Ectatic Diseases describes progression as a change in two or more of the following parameters – steepening of the anterior or posterior corneal surface, or thinning and/or an increase in the rate of corneal thickness change from the periphery to the thinnest point [54]. Contact lenses can distort the cornea and as such need to be discontinued prior to preoperative measurements. Soft contacts should be discontinued for at least 1 week [55] and rigid gas permeable (RGP) lenses should be discontinued for 1–2 weeks for every decade of use [56]. Patients with progressive disease may be candidates for corneal crosslinking (CXL) which has been shown to help strengthen the cornea by forming

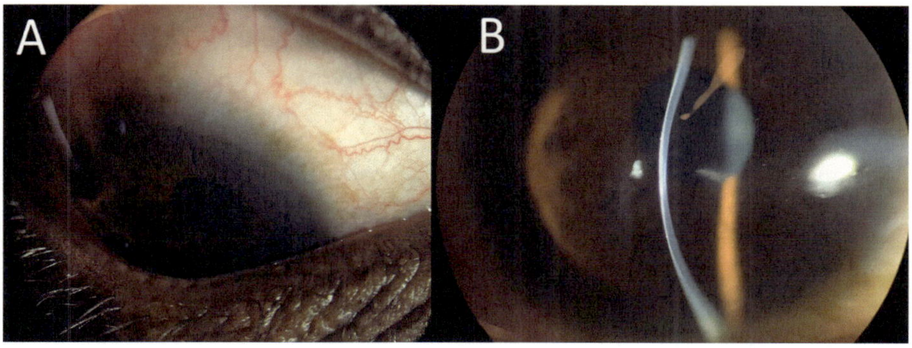

Figure 13.
Slit lamp photograph of an eye with keratoconus demonstrating Munson's sign with V-shaped indentation of the lower eyelid with downgaze (A). Slit beam highlights the apical thinning with ectasia and anterior scarring (B).

new bonds between the collagen fibers in the cornea [57]. As there can be a flattening effect from crosslinking, one should observe for at least 6 months and repeat measurements to document stability prior to cataract surgery. Aiming with a myopic post-refractive goal would be prudent since additional flattening may occur later after the CXL. Additionally, intrastromal corneal ring segment (ICRS) placement has been shown to flatten the cornea. For patients with severe ectatic disease not amenable to contact lenses or with scarring, DALK or PKP can also be effective treatments [58, 59]. Depending on patient goals and surgeon preference, the patient's cataract surgery may have to wait until sutures are removed (starting 3–6 months following surgery) or astigmatism is minimized with selective suture removal. Again, stability of corneal measurements should be documented prior to cataract surgery.

Preoperatively cone location and centration should be evaluated. Patients with central cones tend to be more myopic whereas peripheral cones can actually result in mild hyperopia. Cylinder is affected by both cone location and shape as well [60]. Disease staging helps guide preoperative planning and can be done using the Amsler-Krumeich classification or the newer ABCD classification which has the advantage of staging early and subclinical disease by assessing anterior and posterior radii of curvature from a 3-mm optical zone at the thinnest point of the cornea, minimal corneal thickness, and best spectacle distance visual acuity [61]. One study emphasized the importance of accurately staging keratoconus by showing that using measured K values for IOL selection results in better outcomes in mild to moderate disease while standard K values (43.25) produce better results in severe keratoconus ($K > 55$) [62].

There are several devices available to measure biometry and keratometry. Routine methods using Placido disk based corneal topography devices assess only the anterior surface of the cornea whereas an elevation-based Scheimpflug imaging device will calculate total corneal refractive power by assessing anterior and posterior corneal curvatures [63]. The ratio between anterior and posterior corneal curvature is altered in keratoconus [64] thereby making the Placido disk based corneal topography devices less accurate and may lead to a higher chance of residual hyperopia, especially for advanced Keratoconus [63]. Currently available keratometry and biometry measuring devices include the Pentacam HR and AXL (Oculus GmbH, Wetzlar, Germany), IOL Master 700 (Carl Zeiss Meditec AG, Jena, Germany), Lenstar LS 900 (Haag-Streit AG, Koeniz, Switzerland), Sirius (Costruzione Strumenti Oftalmici, Florence, Italy), and Galilei G6 (Ziemer, Biel, Switzerland). Multiple studies have been conducted comparing these various devices in patients with keratoconus [65–73]. After reviewing the available data comparing these devices, Moshirfar et al. published a paper ultimately recommending obtaining Pentacam measurements, comparing them across more than one device and selecting the measurements that result in the highest calculated IOL power. Doing so reduces the risk of hyperopic surprise postoperatively [56].

As alluded to above, formula selection in patients with keratoconus is challenging as traditional formulas were developed based on a normal eye. Many studies comparing outcomes using different formulas have been done and demonstrate that the best formula may depend on the stage of the patient's disease. The largest case series of cataract surgery in keratoconus looked at a total of 147 eyes and compared the precision of IOL formulas which are used routinely in normal eyes, (Haigis, Barrett Universal 2, Holladay 1 and 2, Hoffer Q, SRK/T, and Kane) compared to IOL formulas which are made exclusively for Keratoconus patients (Kane Keratoconus formula and Holladay 2 with Keratoconus Adjustment). The authors concluded that the Kane Keratoconus formula performed best in all stages of keratoconus followed by SRK/T.

Furthermore, the authors suggested target refractions specific to each Krumeich stage. In stage 1 Keratoconus patients, there should be between no adjustment to −1.0 for the target refraction, for stage 2 a myopic target of −0.75 to −1.5 should be aimed for, and for stage 3 a myopic target of −2.0 to −3.0 [74].

7.2 Intraoperative considerations

A potentially controversial topic is the use of toric IOLs in patients with keratoconus. Their use has been investigated in patients with stable mild to moderate keratoconus. In these patients, toric lenses have shown significant improvement in postoperative uncorrected and best corrected visual acuity without causing significant corneal higher order aberrations [75, 76]. Toric IOLs should not be considered in patients with progressive disease, difficult refraction, or if there is a high difference between preoperative RGP lens corrected visual acuity and spectacle corrected visual acuity [77]. Aspheric IOLs should not be placed in patients with keratoconus as these IOLs are designed to eliminate the positive spherical aberration added by traditional IOLs. Due to the hyperprolate nature of keratoconus eyes, they would experience more negative spherical aberration [78] and worsen the hyperopic refractive shift. If the surgeon believes the patient will need a keratoplasty in the future after cataract surgery has been performed, the presence of a low power IOL will likely worsen hyperopia due to the subsequent loss of corneal power after the transplant. It may be better to perform the keratoplasty and later perform the cataract surgery after a period of stabilization and selective suture removal.

The irregular astigmatism secondary to corneal warpage in keratoconus can lead to intraoperative image distortion making cataract surgery more challenging for the surgeon. Use of RGP lenses intraoperatively can be quite helpful to reduce distortion and improve depth perception [79, 80]. Trypan blue can be helpful for visualization through an ectatic cornea often with scarring.

Incision sites can result in changes to K values and the cataract surgery itself might increase the probability of disease progression [81]. A pachymap can be helpful to guide incision sites to avoid the thinnest areas (avoid the cone/apex) [82]. These incisions should be made near the limbus to avoid surgically induced astigmatism and violation of the thinned, ectactic cornea [83]. Alternatively, a small scleral tunnel can be made if universally thin. Multiple studies have shown that clear corneal incisions are safe and may not necessarily need suturing [75, 84–86]; however, corneal sutures are generally considered more reliable and provide an opportunity for correction of astigmatism and subsequently of best uncorrected visual acuity in some patients [83].

7.3 Postoperative management

Many keratoconus patients will have residual refractive error, particularly those with severe disease. As mentioned previously, IOL calculations can be challenging in keratoconus patients and unsurprisingly postoperative refractive error is common. Spectacles can be used in patients with mild residual error [87] although they cannot correct for irregular astigmatism commonly seen in keratoconus. Soft contact lenses and soft toric lenses can be used in patient's with low refractive error, regular astigmatism or mild irregular astigmatism as the soft contact lens covers the anterior corneal abnormalities [88]. In patients with a more significant refractive error, RGP, piggy-back, hybrid, or scleral contact lenses can be tried [87–90]. Surgical options include IOL exchange, but it should be noted that IOL exchange may have a higher risk of complications [91] and that if attempted, it is advised to perform the lens exchange within 3–6 months after initial IOL implantation due to fibrosis around the IOL [92]. Surgical placement of a secondary IOL is also an option and both anterior chamber iris claw lens and piggyback lenses implanted in the sulcus have been accomplished with satisfactory results [93–98].

8. Conclusion

With the prevalence of ocular surface and corneal conditions, ophthalmologists will commonly encounter cataract surgery in the setting of coexisting corneal disease. This chapter has investigated some of these challenges and the available literature specific to ocular surface disease, corneal opacification, endothelial disease, and keratoconus for a cataract surgeon to consider including preoperative assessment, treatment and diagnostic testing, intraoperative pearls and techniques, and postoperative management to facilitate good surgical outcomes for our patients.

Conflict of interest

Brian Bird has no conflict of interest to declare.

Albert Y. Cheung, MD reports consulting for Sight Sciences, Tarsus, Moya ocular, BrightStar Therapeutics.

John D Sheppard reports consulting for Allergan, AbbVie, Alcon, Aldeyra Therapeutics, Bausch & Lomb, BioTissue, ClarisBio, Dompe, EyeDetec, Eye Point, EyeGate, Fortress Bio, NovaBay, Novartis, Noveome, LayerBio, Mallinckrodt, Mati, Ocular Therapeutix, Kala, RPS, Tarsier, Tearlab, Johnson & Johnson, Fidia, Clarios, Visus, Topivert, Noveome, Oyster Point, Santen, Sun Pharmaceutical Industries, Eyevance, ScienceBased Health, and Quidel; and ownership interest in ClarisBio, Noveome, EyeDetec, EyeRx Pharma, Oyster Point, RPS, TearLab, EyeGate, Strathspey Crowne, Mati, and CVP Partners.

Author details

Brian A. Bird[1*], Albert Y. Cheung[1,2] and John D. Sheppard[1,2]

1 Eastern Virginia Medical School, Norfolk VA, USA

2 Virginia Eye Consultants, Norfolk VA, USA

*Address all correspondence to: brianbird43@gmail.com

References

[1] GBD 2019 Blindness and Vision Impairment Collaborators; Vision Loss Expert Group of the Global Burden of Disease Study. Causes of blindness and vision impairment in 2020 and trends over 30 years, and prevalence of avoidable blindness in relation to VISION 2020: The right to sight: An analysis for the global burden of disease study. The Lancet Global Health. 2021;**9**(2):e144-e160. DOI: 10.1016/S2214-109X(20)30489-7 Epub 2020 Dec 1. Erratum in: Lancet Glob Health. 2021;9(4):e408

[2] Mason L, Jafri S, Dortonne I, Sheppard JD Jr. Emerging therapies for dry eye disease. Expert Opinion on Emerging Drugs. 2021;**26**(4):401-413. DOI: 10.1080/14728214.2021.2011858 Epub 2021 Dec 7

[3] Rouen PA, White ML. Dry eye disease. Home Healthcare Now. 2018;**36**(2):74-83

[4] Basic and clinical science course. Orbit, eyelids, and lacrimal system. American Academy of Ophthalmology. 2012;**7**:243-244

[5] Epitropoulos AT, Matossian C, Berdy GJ, Malhotra RP, Potvin R. Effect of tear osmolarity on repeatability of keratometry for cataract surgery planning. Journal of Cataract and Refractive Surgery. 2015;**41**:1672-1677

[6] Pucker AD, Ng SM, Nichols JJ. Over the counter (OTC) artificial tear drops for dry eye syndrome. Cochrane Database of Systematic Reviews. 2016;**2**:CD009729

[7] Sall K, Stevenson OD, Mundorf TK, et al. Two multicenter, randomized studies of the efficacy and safety of cyclosporine ophthalmic emulsion in moderate to severe dry eye disease. CsA phase 3 study group. Ophthalmology. 2000;**107**(4):631-639

[8] Highlights of Prescribing Information [Internet]. cequapro. 2019. Available from: https://cequapro.com/pdf/CequaPI.pdf [Accessed: June 23, 2021].

[9] De Paiva CS, Pflugfelder SC, Ng SM, et al. Topical cyclosporine a therapy for dry eye syndrome. Cochrane Database of Systematic Reviews. 2019;**9**(9):CD010051

[10] Donnenfeld ED, Solomon R, Roberts CW, et al. Cyclosporine 0.05% to improve visual outcomes after multifocal intraocular lens implantation. Journal of Cataract and Refractive Surgery. 2010;**36**:1095-1100

[11] Liu Y, Kam WR, Ding J, Sullivan DA. One man's poison is another man's meat. Using azithromycin- induced phospholipidosis to promote ocular surface health. Toxicology. 2014;**320**:1-5

[12] Zhao Y, Veerappan A, Yeo S, Rooney DM, Acharya RU, Tan JH, et al. Clinical trial of thermal pulsation (LipiFlow) in meibomian gland dysfunction with pretreatment meibography. Eye & Contact Lens. 2016;**42**:339

[13] Hagen KB, Bedi R, Blackie CA, Christenson-Akagi KJ. Comparison of a single-dose vectored thermal pulsation procedure with a 3-month course of daily oral doxycycline for moderate-to-severe meibomian gland dysfunction. Clinical Ophthalmology (Auckl, NZ). 2018;**12**:161

[14] Craig JP, Chen YH, Turnbull PR. Prospective trial of intense pulsed light for the treatment of meibomian gland dysfunction. Investigative

Ophthalmology & Visual Science. 2015;**56**:1965-1970

[15] Arita R, Fukuoka S, Morishige N. Therapeutic efficacy of intense pulsed light in patients with refractory meibomian gland dysfunction. The Ocular Surface. 2019;**17**:104-110

[16] Rong B, Tang Y, Tu P, et al. Intense pulsed light applied directly on eyelids combined with meibomian gland expression to treat meibomian gland dysfunction. Photomedicine and Laser Surgery. 2018;**36**:326-332

[17] Oxervate full prescribing information [Internet]. oxervate-approved. 2019. Available from: https://oxervate-approved.com/wp-content/uploads/2020/05/OXERVATE-USPI.pdf [Accessed: June 23, 2021]

[18] Pflugfelder SC, Massaro-Giordano M, Perez VL, et al. Topical recombinant human nerve growth factor (Cenegermin) for neurotrophic keratopathy: A multicenter randomized vehicle-controlled pivotal trial. Ophthalmology. 2020;**127**(1):14-26

[19] Geerling G, Dart JKG. Management and outcome of cataract surgery in ocular cicatricial pemphigoid. Graefe's Archive for Clinical and Experimental Ophthalmology. 2000;**238**:112-118

[20] Sangwan VS, Burman S. Cataract surgery in Stevens–Johnson syndrome. Journal of Cataract and Refractive Surgery. 2005;**31**:860-862

[21] Perez VL, Azar DT, Foster CS. Sterile corneal melting and necrotizing scleritis after cataract surgery in patients with rheumatoid arthritis and collagen vascular disease. Seminars in Ophthalmology. 2002;**17**:124-130

[22] Sangwan VS, Surender P, Burman S. Cataract surgery in patients with Mooren's ulcer. Journal of Cataract and Refractive Surgery. 2005;**31**:359-362

[23] Kim SW, Park S, Im CY, Seo KY, Kim EK. Prediction of mean corneal power change after pterygium excision. Cornea. 2014;**33**:148-153

[24] Sharma B et al. Refractive outcomes of simultaneous pterygium and cataract surgery with fibrin glue. Cureus. 2021;**13**(11):e19857

[25] Kamiya K et al. Predictability of intraocular lens power calculation after simultaneous pterygium excision and cataract surgery. Medicine. 2015;**94**(52):e2232

[26] Nejima R, Masuda A, Minami K, Mori Y, Hasegawa Y, Miyata K. Topographic changes after excision surgery of primary pterygia and the effect of pterygium size on topograpic restoration. Eye & Contact Lens. 2015;**41**:58-63

[27] Pujari A, Sharma N. The emerging role of anterior segment optical coherence tomography in cataract surgery: Current role and future perspectives. Clinical Ophthalmology. 2021;**15**:389-401. DOI: 10.2147/OPTH.S286996

[28] Tabatabaei SA, Soleimani M, Etesali H, Naderan M. Accuracy of swept source optical coherence tomography and ultrasound biomicroscopy for evaluation of posterior lens capsule in traumatic cataract. American Journal of Ophthalmology. 2020;**20**:30141. DOI: 10.1016/j.ajo.2020.03.030

[29] Bae SS, Chan CC. Superficial keratectomy: Indications and outcomes. Canadian Journal of Ophthalmology. 2018;**53**(6):553-559. DOI: 10.1016/j.jcjo.2018.01.030 Epub 2018 Apr 4

[30] Goerlitz-Jessen MF, Gupta PK, Kim T. Impact of epithelial basement membrane dystrophy and Salzmann nodular degeneration on biometry measurements. Journal of Cataract and Refractive Surgery. 2019;**45**(8):1119-1123. DOI: 10.1016/j.jcrs.2019.03.014 Epub 2019 Jun 4

[31] Ayres BD, Rapuano CJ. Excimer laser phototherapeutic keratectomy. The Ocular Surface. 2006;**4**(4):196-206. DOI: 10.1016/s1542-0124(12)70166-0

[32] Deshmukh R, Reddy JC, Rapuano CJ, Vaddavalli PK. Phototherapeutickeratectomy:Indications, methods and decision making. Indian Journal of Ophthalmology. 2020;**68**(12):2856-2866. DOI: 10.4103/ijo.IJO_1524_20

[33] Pereira-Souza AL, Ambrósio R Jr, Bandeira F, Salomão MQ, Souza Lima A, Wilson SE. Topical losartan for treating corneal fibrosis (haze): First clinical experience. Journal of Refractive Surgery. 2022;**38**(11):741-746

[34] Norn MS. Preoperative trypan blue vital staining of corneal endothelium; eight years' follow-up. Acta Ophthalmologica. 1908;**58**:550-555

[35] Sinha R, Sharma N, Vajpayee RB. Visual outcome of cataract surgery with pupillary sphincterotomy in eyes with coexisting corneal opacity. BMC Medicine. 2004;**7**(2):10

[36] Nishimura A, Kobayashi A, Segawa Y, Sugiyama K. Endoillumination-assisted cataract surgery in a patient with corneal opacity. Journal of Cataract and Refractive Surgery. 2003;**29**(12):2277-2280

[37] Oshima Y, Shima C, Maeda N, Tano Y. Chandelier retroillumination-assisted torsional oscillation for cataract surgery in patients with severe corneal opacity. Journal of Cataract and Refractive Surgery. 2007;**33**(12):2018-2022

[38] Shimmura S, Ohashi Y, Shiroma H, Shimazaki J, Tsubota K. Corneal opacity and cataract: Triple procedure versus secondary approach. Cornea. 2003;**22**:234-238

[39] Javadi MA, Feizi S, Moein HR. Simultaneous penetrating keratoplasty and cataract surgery. Journal of Ophthalmic and Vision Research. 2013;**8**:39-46

[40] Davis EA, Azar DT, Jakobs FM, Stark WJ. Refractive and keratometric results after the triple procedure. Ophthalmology. 1998;**105**:624-630

[41] Bersudsky V, Rehany U, Rumelt S. Risk factors for failure of simultaneous penetrating keratoplasty and cataract extraction. Journal of Cataract and Refractive Surgery. 2004;**30**:1940-1947

[42] Binder PS. Intraocular lens powers used in the triple procedure. Effect on visual acuity and refractive error. Ophthalmology. 1985;**92**:1561-1566

[43] Geggel HS. Intraocular lens implantation after penetrating keratoplasty improved unaided visual acuity, astigmatism, and safety in patients with combined corneal disease and cataract. Ophthalmology. 1990;**97**:1460-1467

[44] Hayashi K, Yoshida M, Manabe S, Hirata A. Cataract surgery in eyes with low corneal endothelial cell density. Journal of Cataract and Refractive Surgery. 2011;**37**:1419-1425

[45] Sun SY, Wacker K, Baratz KH, Patel SV. Determining subclinical edema in Fuchs endothelial corneal dystrophy:

Revised classification using Scheimpflug tomography for preoperative assessment. Ophthalmology. 2019;**126**(2):195-204

[46] Patel SV et al. Predicting the prognosis of Fuchs endothelial corneal dystrophy by using Scheimpflug tomography. Ophthalmology. 2020;**127**(3):315-323

[47] Walkow T, Anders N, Klebe S. Endothelial cell loss after phacoemulsification: Relation to preoperative and intraoperative parameters. Journal of Cataract and Refractive Surgery. 2000;**26**:727-732

[48] Hugod M, Storr-Paulsen A, Norregaard J, et al. Corneal endothelial cell changes associated with cataract surgery in patients with type 2 diabetes mellitus. Cornea. 2011;**30**:749-753

[49] Rabinowitz YS. Keratoconus. Survey of Ophthalmology. 1998;**42**(4):297-319. DOI: 10.1016/S0039-6257(97)00119-7

[50] Krachmer JH, Feder RS, Belin MW. Keratoconus and related noninflammatory corneal thinning disorders. Survey of Ophthalmology. 1984;**28**(4):293-322. DOI: 10.1016/0039-6257(84)90094-8

[51] Romero-Jiménez M, Santodomingo-Rubido J, Wolffsohn JS. Keratoconus: A review. Contact Lens Anterior Eye. 2010;**33**(4):157-166. DOI: 10.1016/j.clae.2010.04.006

[52] Thebpatiphat N, Hammersmith KM, Rapuano CJ, Ayres BD, Cohen EJ. Cataract surgery in keratoconus. Eye & Contact Lens. 2007;**33**(5):244-246. DOI: 10.1097/ICL.0b013e318030c96d

[53] Ghiasian L, Abolfathzadeh N, Manafi N, Hadavandkhani A. Intraocular lens power calculation in keratoconus; a review of literature. Journal of Current Ophthalmology. 2019;**31**:127-134

[54] Gomes JAP, Tan D, Rapuano CJ, et al. Global consensus on keratoconus and ectatic diseases. Cornea. 2015;**34**:359-369

[55] Budak K, Hamed AM, Friedman NJ, Koch DD. Preoperative screening of contact lens wearers before refractive surgery. Journal of Cataract and Refractive Surgery. 1999;**25**:1080-1086

[56] Moshirfar M, Ziari M, Ronquillo YC. Cataract surgery considerations in patients with prior history of keratoconus and ectasia. Current Opinion in Ophthalmology. 2023;**34**(1):41-47. DOI: 10.1097/ICU.0000000000000908 Epub 2022 Sep 19

[57] Zaky AG, Khalaf Allah MT, Sarhan AE. Combined corneal cross-linking and 3208 intrastromal corneal ring segments in progressive keratoconus: One-year results. Graefe's Archive for Clinical and Experimental Ophthalmology. 2020;**258**:2441-2447

[58] Sutton G, Hodge C, Mcghee CNJ. Rapid visual recovery after penetrating keratoplasty for keratoconus. Clinical & Experimental Ophthalmology. 2008;**36**:725-730

[59] Feizi S, Javadi MA, Kheiri B. Effect of keratoconus severity on clinical outcomes after deep anterior lamellar keratoplasty. American Journal of Ophthalmology. 2019;**202**:15-22

[60] Eliasy A, Abass A, Lopes BT, et al. Characterization of cone size and centre in keratoconic corneas. Journal of the Royal Society Interface. 2020;**17**:20200271

[61] Belin MW, Kundu G, Shetty N, et al. ABCD: A new classification for keratoconus. Indian Journal of Ophthalmology. 2020;**68**:2831-2834

[62] Watson MP, Anand S, Bhogal M, et al. Cataract surgery outcome in eyes with keratoconus. The British Journal of Ophthalmology. 2014;**98**:361-364

[63] Wang KM, Jun AS, Ladas JG, Siddiqui AA, Woreta F, Srikumaran D. Accuracy of intraocular lens formulas in eyes with keratoconus. American Journal of Ophthalmology. 2020;**212**:26-33. DOI: 10.1016/j.ajo. 2019.11.019

[64] Tomidokoro A, Oshika T, Amano S, Higaki S, Maeda N, Miyata K. Changes in anterior and posterior corneal curvatures in keratoconus. Ophthalmology. 2000;**107**(7):1328-1332. DOI: 10.1016/S0161-6420(00)00159-7

[65] Kamiya K, Iijima K, Nobuyuki S, et al. Predictability of intraocular lens power calculation for cataract with keratoconus: A multicenter study. Scientific Reports. 2018;**8**(1):1-7. DOI: 10.1038/s41598-018-20040-w

[66] Chalkiadaki E, Gartaganis PS, Ntravalias T, et al. Agreement in anterior segment measurements between swept-source and Scheimpflug-based optical biometries in keratoconic eyes: A pilot study. Therapeutic Advances in Ophthalmology. 2022;**14**:25158414211063283 The study compares the agreement of Scheimpflug based biometry devices

[67] Kim J, Whang W-J, Kim H-S. Analysis of total corneal astigmatism with a rotating Scheimpflug camera in keratoconus. BMC Ophthalmology. 2020;**20**:475

[68] Saglik A, Celik H. Comparison of Holladay equivalent keratometry readings and anterior corneal surface keratometry measurements in keratoconus. International Ophthalmology. 2019;**39**:1501-1509

[69] Güçlü H, Akaray I, Kaya S, et al. Agreement of anterior segment parameters between schiempflug topography and swept-source optic coherence based optic biometry in keratoconus and healthy subjects. Eye & Contact Lens. 2021;**47**:539-545

[70] Altınel MG, Uslu H. Agreement of keratometric readings measured using rotating Scheimpflug imaging, auto-refractokeratometer, and biograph in eyes with keratoconus. International Ophthalmology. 2021;**41**:1659-1669

[71] Moshirfar M, Tenney S, McCabe S, Schmid G. Repeatability and reproducibility of the galilei G6 and its agreement with the pentacam1 AXL in optical biometry and corneal tomography. Expert Review of Medical Devices. 2022;**19**:375-383

[72] Shetty R, Arora V, Jayadev C, et al. Repeatability and agreement of three scheimpflug-based imaging systems for measuring anterior segment parameters in keratoconus. Investigative Ophthalmology & Visual Science. 2014;**55**:5263-5268

[73] Meyer JJ, Gokul A, Vellara HR, et al. Repeatability and agreement of orbscan II, pentacam HR, and galilei tomography systems in corneas with keratoconus. American Journal of Ophthalmology. 2017;**175**:122-128

[74] Kane JX, Connell B, Yip H, et al. Accuracy of intraocular lens power formulas modified for patients with keratoconus. Ophthalmology. 2020;**127**(8):1037-1042. DOI: 10.1016/j.ophtha.2020.02.008

[75] Hashemi H, Heidarian S, Seyedian MA, Yekta A, Khabazkhoob M. Evaluation of the results of using toric IOL in the cataract surgery of keratoconus patients. Eye & Contact

Lens. 2015;**41**(6):354-358. DOI: 10.1097/ICL.0000000000000136

[76] Nanavaty MA, Lake DB, Daya SM. Outcomes of pseudophakic toric intraocular lens implantation in keratoconic eyes with cataract. Journal of Refractive Surgery. 2012;**28**(12):884-890. DOI: 10.3928/1081597X-20121106-02

[77] Navas A, Suárez R. One-year follow-up of toric intraocular lens implantation in forme fruste keratoconus. Journal of Cataract and Refractive Surgery. 2009;**35**(11):2024-2027. DOI: 10.1016/j.jcrs.2009.05.043

[78] Savini G, Barboni P, Carbonelli M, Hoffer KJ. Repeatability of automatic measurements by a new Scheimpflug camera combined with Placido topography. Journal of Cataract and Refractive Surgery. 2011;**37**:1809-1816

[79] Oie Y, Kamei M, Matsumura N, et al. Rigid gas-permeable contact lens–assisted cataract surgery in patients with severe keratoconus. Journal of Cataract and Refractive Surgery. 2014;**40**(3):345-348. DOI: 10.1016/j.jcrs.2014.01.001

[80] Chanbour W, Harb F, Jarade E. A modified customized rigid gas permeable contact lens to improve visualization during phacoemulsification in ectatic corneas. Medical Hypothesis Discovery and Innovation in Ophthalmology. 2020;**9**(1):1

[81] Bourges J-L. Cataract surgery in keratoconus with irregular astigmatism. In: Astigmatism-Optics, Physio Manage Croatia Tech. Intech Open; 29 Feb 2012. 320 p. DOI: 10.5772/759. ISBN: 978-953-51-0230-4. EBOOK (PDF) ISBN: 978-953-51-6874-4

[82] Aiello F, Nasser Q, Nucci C, et al. Cataract surgery in patients with keratoconus: Pearls and pitfalls. The Open Ophthalmology Journal. 2017;**11**:194

[83] Hashemi H, Khabazkhoob M, Soroush S, et al. The location of incision in cataract surgery and its impact on induced astigmatism. Current Opinion in Ophthalmology. 2016;**27**:58-64

[84] Kamiya K, Shimizu K, Miyake T. Changes in astigmatism and corneal higher-order aberrations after phacoemulsification with toric intraocular lens implantation for mild keratoconus with cataract. Japanese Journal of Ophthalmology. 2016;**60**(4):302-308. DOI: 10.1007/s10384-016-0449-x

[85] Alió JL, Peña-García P, Guliyeva FA, Soria FA, Zein G, Abu Mustafa SK. MICS with toric intraocular lenses in keratoconus: Outcomes and predictability analysis of postoperative refraction. British Journal of Ophthalmology. 2014;**98**(3):365-370. DOI: 10.1136/bjophthal mol-2013-303765

[86] Alfonso JF, Lisa C, Cueto LF-V, Poo-López A, Madrid-Costa D, Fernández-Vega L. Sequential intrastromal corneal ring segment and monofocal intraocular lens implantation for keratoconus and cataract: Long-term follow-up. Journal of Cataract and Refractive Surgery. 2017;**43**(2):246-254. DOI: 10.1016/j.jcrs.2016.11.044

[87] Andreanos KD, Hashemi K, Petrelli M, Droutsas K, Georgalas I, Kymionis GD. Keratoconus treatment algorithm. Ophthalmology and Therapy. 2017;**6**(2):245-262. DOI: 10.1007/s40123-017-0099-1

[88] Katsoulos C, Karageorgiadis L, Vasileiou N, Mousafeiropoulos T, Asimellis G. Customized hydrogel contact lenses for keratoconus

incorporating correction for vertical coma aberration. Ophthalmic & Physiological Optics. 2009;**29**(3):321-329. DOI: 10.1111/j.1475-1313.2009.00645.x

[89] Rathi VM, Mandathara PS, Dumpati S. Contact lens in keratoconus. Indian Journal of Ophthalmology. 2013;**61**(8):410. DOI: 10.4103/0301-4738.116066

[90] Picot C, Gauthier A, Campolmi N, Delbosc B. Quality of life in patients wearing scleral lenses. The Journal Français d'Ophtalmologie. 2015;**38**(7):615-619. DOI: 10.1016/j.jfo.2014.10.018

[91] Mamalis N, Brubaker J, Davis D, Espandar L, Werner L. Complications of foldable intraocular lenses requiring explantation or secondary intervention—2007 survey update. Journal of Cataract and Refractive Surgery. 2008;**34**(9):1584-1591. DOI: 10.1016/j.jcrs.2008.05.046

[92] Leysen I, Bartholomeeusen E, Coeckelbergh T, Tassignon M-JB. Surgical outcomes of intraocular lens exchange: Five-year study. Journal of Cataract and Refractive Surgery. 2009;**35**(6):1013-1018. DOI: 10.1016/j.jcrs.2009.01.024

[93] Oshika T, Inamura M, Inoue Y, et al. Incidence and outcomes of repositioning surgery to correct misalignment of toric intraocular lenses. Ophthalmology. 2018;**125**(1):31-35. DOI: 10.1016/j.ophtha.2017.07.004

[94] Budo C, Bartels MC, van Rij G. Implantation of artisan toric phakic intraocular lenses for the correction of astigmatism and spherical errors in patients with keratoconus. Journal of Refractive Surgery. 2005;**21**(3):218-222

[95] Moshirfar M, Grégoire FJ, Mirzaian G, Whitehead GF, Kang PC. Use of Verisyse iris-supported phakic intraocular lens for myopia in keratoconic patients. Journal of Cataract and Refractive Surgery. 2006;**32**(7):1227-1232. DOI: 10.1016/j.jcrs.2006.02.017

[96] Fernández-Vega Cueto L, Lisa C, Poo-López A, Madrid-Costa D, Merayo-Lloves J, Alfonso JF. Intrastromal corneal ring segment implantation in 409 paracentral keratoconic eyes. Cornea. 2016;**35**(11):1421-1426. DOI: 10.1097/ICO.0000000000000978

[97] Sedaghat M, Ansari-Astaneh M-R, Zarei-Ghanavati M, Davis SW, Sikder S. Artisan iris-supported phakic IOL implantation in patients with keratoconus: A review of 16 eyes. Journal of Refractive Surgery. 2011;**27**(7):489-493. DOI: 10.3928/1081597X-20110203-01

[98] Alfonso JF. Myopic phakic STAAR collamer posterior chamber intraocular lenses for keratoconus. Journal of Refractive Surgery. 2008;**24**(9):867

Chapter 3

Cataract Surgery and Dry Eye

Kenneth Gek-Jin Ooi, King Fai Calvin Leung, Jessica Xiong, Pauline Khoo and Stephanie Louise Watson

Abstract

This chapter outlines preoperative, intraoperative, and postoperative considerations with respect to dry eye (DE) and its impact on cataract surgery, to guide optimization of patient satisfaction with their refractive outcomes. A systematic review was performed and reported according to the Preferred Reporting Items for Systematic Reviews and Meta-Analyses (PRISMA) statement. MEDLINE (Ovid), EMBASE (Ovid), Cochrane Library, PubMed, and Scopus, from the date of inception (1946) until 3rd June 2023, were searched. Dry eye and ametropia are among the most common causes of dissatisfaction after cataract surgery and also the most amenable to successful conservative management. Dry eye can reduce contrast sensitivity and increase dysphotopsias in multifocal intraocular lens patients. Several pathophysiological changes occur during and after surgery that influence DE manifestation postoperatively. Dry eye symptoms and signs generally normalize at around 3 months in both normal and DE patients, but a significant minority have ongoing discomfort. A number of systemic and ocular conditions are identified, which may aid in preoperative risk evaluation. Preoperative symptom evaluation, examination, and investigation techniques are also summarized and their influence on refractive outcomes emphasized. Current preoperative, intraoperative, and postoperative measures to decrease burden are additionally evaluated.

Keywords: cataract surgery, dry eye, meibomian gland dysfunction, blepharitis, intraocular lens

1. Introduction

Cataracts and dry eye (DE) are both age-related conditions underpinned by increased oxidative stress with time and commonly presenting to clinicians [1–3]. Cataract surgery rates are increasing, and postoperative outcomes are improving worldwide [4, 5]. As the world's population is forecasted to increase life expectancy by 4.4 years by 2040 for both men and women [6], and as we are becoming more adept at defining and diagnosing dry eye [7, 8], DE reporting rates are also expected to increase. Both cataracts and DE are associated with impaired vision [4, 9]. While rapid postoperative visual recovery is possible [4], with good visual outcomes in DE patients [10], surgery may lead to DE development or worsening [11]. This review focuses on pre-, intra-, and postoperative factors that clinicians can consider to optimize refractive outcomes in DE patients.

2. Impact

The pre-corneal tear film is the first refractive plane, and interference leads to unfavorable postoperative refractive results impacting satisfaction [12]. Patients may also have eye fatigue and foreign body sensation. This may lead to preserved artificial tear substitute overuse with resultant epithelial toxicity [13] and vicious DE cycle perpetuation.

Dissatisfaction with multifocal Intraocular lenses (IOLs) in particular can result in explantation [14]. Multifocality requires neuroadaptation to adjust to the change in the quality of the retinal image resultant from induced light energy dispersion [12]. Multifocal IOLs are associated with increased dysphotopsia and decreased contrast sensitivity compared with monofocal IOLs [12, 15, 16], as well as increased intraocular stray light [17]. As DE is associated with decreased contrast sensitivity [18], postoperative patients with DE may encounter compounded loss of contrast sensitivity. This can be especially debilitating in mesopic or scotopic conditions [12]. These patients also have increased dysphotopsia after multifocal IOL implantation [12, 13]. The most identifiable causes of multifocal IOL dissatisfaction are residual refractive error and DE with both as the most frequent concurrent complaints [19, 20].

3. Methods

A systematic review was performed and reported according to the Preferred Reporting Items for Systematic Reviews and Meta-Analyses (PRISMA) statement. The following electronic databases were searched: MEDLINE (Ovid), EMBASE (Ovid), Cochrane Library, PubMed, and Scopus, from the date of inception (1946) until 3rd December 2020. The keywords and Medical Subject Headings (MeSH) used were cataract extraction, cataract, phacoemulsification, dry eye, dry eye syndrome, and keratoconjunctivitis sicca.

Duplicates were identified and removed with EndNote (version X9.3.3, Thomson Reuter, New York, USA). A two-stage process was used to identify eligible articles. First, two review authors (K.O. and P.K.) independently evaluated the titles and abstracts. The second stage involved obtaining full-text articles (for available studies) to assess its eligibility. This was independently assessed by K.O. and P.K. Cited articles identified from the search were also reviewed. Disagreements were resolved by discussion. Studies were included if they were full-text articles published about dry eye from cataract surgery. Reviews and editorials and publications not in English were excluded. Reference lists from the studies identified were also reviewed to identify any potential articles missed on the initial search (**Figure 1**).

4. Epidemiology

Globally, a number of cross-sectional studies have investigated dry eye as a comorbidity of cataracts and cataract surgery as a risk factor for worsened dry eye [21–25]. Preoperatively, in a prospective, multicenter, observational 136-patient study (68 males; mean age 70.7 ± 7.8 years) scheduled to undergo surgery, DE incidence was 75.1%; 62.9% had tear breakup times (TBUT) of ≤5 seconds; 77% had positive corneal fluorescein staining (CFS), and 18% had Schirmer's test (ST) with anesthesia (ST-1) ≤ 5 mm. As only 25.9% had a prior DE diagnosis, it was concluded that real-world

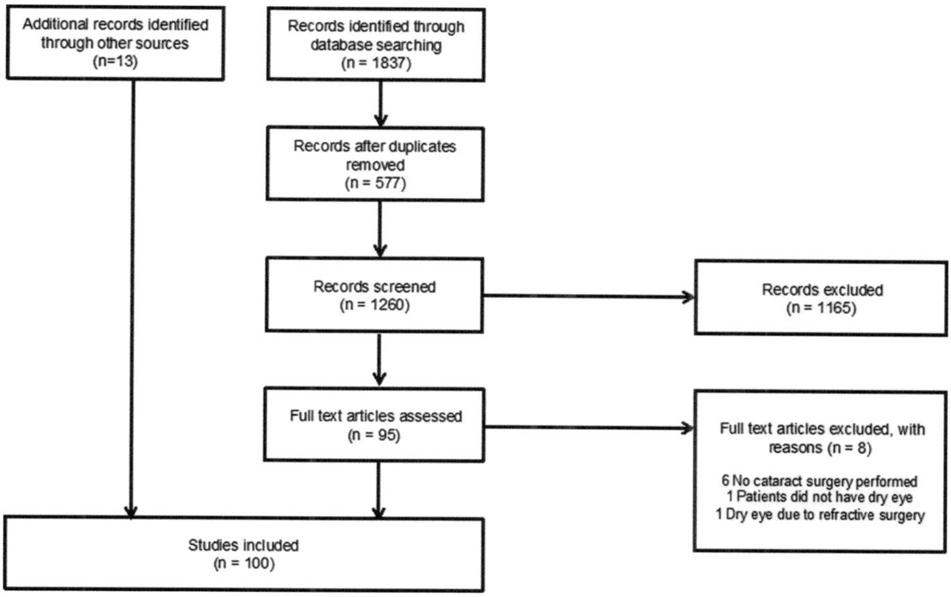

Figure 1.
PRISMA diagram summarizing the study selection process.

setting incidence is higher than anticipated [26]. Similarly, in a study of 342 eyes, it was concluded that the 52% incidence of Meibomian gland (MG) dysfunction (MGD) was high in patients presenting for surgery with correlating lower lipid layer thickness ($P < .05$) and 56% having MG atrophy ≥ Arita grade 1.

One-week postoperatively in 92 patients (31 males; mean age 67.22 ± 8.26 years), DE incidence was 9.8% (95% confidence interval [CI]; 3.6–16.0%), 68.4% (95% CI; 52.9–83.9%) had TBUTs <10 seconds, and 11.9% (95% CI; 3.6–16.0%) had ≤10 mm of ST without anesthesia (ST-2). No correlations were found between postoperative DE and sex ($P = .26$) or age ($P = .17$) [11]. In 54 patients (14 males; mean age 68.02 ± 8.67 years) with monofocal IOLs, postoperative TBUT was reported lower at 2 months in dissatisfied (n = 27) patients at 5.4 ± 2.7 seconds as compared to those who were satisfied (n = 27) at 6.9 ± 3.0 seconds ($P < .045$). Visual Function Index −14, Ocular Surface Disease Index (OSDI), and Shortened Health Anxiety Inventory scores were also worse in the unsatisfied group ($P < .002$) [27].

At 3 months, postoperative incidence of increased OSDI scores at week one (65.5) became normalized (14.1), comparable to preoperatively (10.5) in a 96-patient cohort (35 males; mean age of 63.1 ± 8.3 years). Week one TBUTs were 8.7 ± 0.48 ($P < .001$) seconds and improved to 14.3 ± 0.37 seconds at 3 months, comparable to preoperatively at 15.8 ± 0.31 seconds ($P = .089$). Baseline ST-1 of 24.5 ± 0.59 mm worsened at week one to 15.2 ± 0.64 seconds ($P < .001$) and trended toward baseline at 3 months but were still reduced at 21.8 ± 0.64 seconds ($P < .001$) [28]. Kasetsuwan et al. also reported mean OSDI scores (17.34) improvement and Oxford ocular surface staining (Grade 1) at 3 months returning toward baseline (12.57 and Grade 1, respectively) [11]. At 3 months, however, mean ST-1 and TBUT also reduced (9.83 mm, 5.11 seconds, respectively) compared to baseline (14.14 mm, 12.15 seconds, respectively) [11].

At a mean of 2.1 ± 3.4 years (0.5–21 years) postoperatively, corneal epitheliopathy frequencies in controls who had no cataracts (n = 1225) and patients who had cataract extraction in both eyes (n = 172) were 11% and 16.5% (P = .008). There was also a 57% increased prevalence of severe keratoconjunctivitis in pseudophakes compared to controls (P = .02). Among DE symptoms, sensitivity to bright light was different between cases and controls; multivariable-adjusted OR (95% CI) comparing pseudophakes with non-cataract patients was 0.56 (0.34–0.92) (P = .02). There was, however, a difference in mean age in years (SD) between controls and surgery patients at 65.4 (9.1) versus 75.4 (9.0) at P < .001 [29].

In 96 chronic DE patients (30 males; mean age 68.46 ± 8.14 years) at 3 months, it was reported that OSDI also increased postoperatively but returned to preoperative levels at 3 months [30]. Oxford scale CFS worsened but improved and resembled preoperative patterns at 3 months. Similar worsening occurred for TBUT and ST-1, but these also returned to baseline at 3 months (P = .078 and P = .748) and remained not different at 2 years (P = .124 and P = .214) [30].

5. Pathophysiological changes

5.1 Tears

In 30 patients, TBUT as well as MG expressibility worsened at 1 and 3 months (P < .05) [31]. Han et al. also demonstrated reductions in MG expressibility in their study of 48 patients at 1 and 3 months (P = .016), but no change in optical coherence tomography tear film meniscus height (TMH), depth, and area at 1 and 3 months was recorded (all P values > .05) [32]. One-week keratograph-measured TMH reductions also normalized at 3 months [33]. At 3 months, TBUT normalized to baseline in 19 normal patients after post-op therapy cessation but worsened in 48 with dry eye [34].

In a 34-patient cohort, meibum quality was scored by digital pressure over 8 MGs of the lower lids. Meibum secretion was graded as: 0, clear; 1, cloudy; 2, cloudy with granular debris; and 3, thick like toothpaste. Meibum quality was significantly worse in the DE group than in the no DE group at 1 month (2.9 ± 0.3, 0.5 ± 0.1, respectively) and 2 months postoperatively (3.5 ± 0.5, 0.5 ± 0.1, respectively) (P < .05, respectively) [35]. These results are partially consistent with our own findings at 1 month of a trend toward significance for worsening of meibum quality in MGD patients (Grade 2 versus grade 1, P = .079). We observed our non-MGD patients, however, to worsen from grade 0 (IQR 0-2) at baseline to grade 1 (IQR 0-1.3), P = .024 (Unpublished data).

One month interferometry lipid layer thickness was significantly thinner than at baseline (P = .004) in a 43-patient study. Lipid layer thickness was positively correlated with TBUT (r = .29, P < .001), while OSDI (r = −.38, P < .001), Oxford staining scores (r = −.30, P = .001), and meibum quality (r = −.21, P = .01) were negatively correlated [36]. Significantly increased thinning in cataract surgery patients of greater than 10 years of diabetic duration has also been noted at 1 month postoperatively.

Tear osmolarity at 1 week (n = 37) was shown to increase to 311.8 ± 14.85 mOsm/L as compared to fellow unoperated control eyes, which averaged 301.7 ± 11.84 mOsm/L (P = .013). After 1 month, study group tear osmolarity values decreased to control levels (P > .05) [37]. Gonzales-Mesa et al. have observed patients with preoperative tear osmolarity values of 312 mOsm/L or higher as more likely to have ocular discomfort postoperatively with worsened OSDI compared to those with less than 312 mOsm/L preoperatively (10.37 ± 11.11 versus 16.48 ± 8.08) at 3 months (P = .01) [38].

Tear-film decreases in multiplex assayed IL-1beta, IL-6, MCP-1, TNF-alpha, and IFN-gamma at 1 and 2 months postoperatively are reported as compared to day 1 elevations ($P < .05$, respectively). Corneal staining score was positively correlated, while TBUT was inversely correlated with IL-8, IL-6, IL-1beta, IFN-gamma, TNF-alpha, and MCP-1 concentrations at 1 month. One-month ST-1 scores inversely correlated with IL-6. The authors ascribed cytokines reductions to steroids and antibiotics usage [35]. Decreases in electrolytes, proteins, and mucins, represented as a significant decrease in tear ferning, have also been documented postoperatively [39].

5.2 Eyelid

At 1 and 3 months, Han et al. noted increased lid margin hyperemia ($P < .001$ and $P < .001$, respectively) as well as increased MG orifice plugging ($P = .007$ and $P < .001$, respectively). No exact mechanism is proposed, but ocular surface inflammation itself related to surgery and reduced blink rates from decreased corneal sensation, topical medications, or lid speculum usage lid dysfunction could contribute [32]. In 57 MGD patients, increased lid margin hyperemia and edge swelling was also sustained at 1 month ($P < .05$). Reduced MG expression correlated until Day 14 ($P < .05$) but returned to baseline at 1 month [40].

In our 20-patient cohort at 1 month, infrared meibography revealed no overall MG dropout change as quantified by meiboscore for both MGD ($n = 10$) and non-MGD ($n = 10$) patients compared to baseline (Unpublished data), which is consistent with the findings of Han et al. [32]. Park et al. also described no significant change in meiboscore, but MG changes were seen postoperatively, including gland dropout, shortening, distortion, and proximal dilation [35]. On meibography, upper lid MG loss is reported to be significantly higher at 1 and 3 months compared to preoperatively with a correlation between upper lid MG loss and OSDI score at 1 month ($R = 0.37$; $P = .05$) [31].

5.3 Conjunctiva

Reduced goblet cell density (GCD) is reported by impression cytology in a prospective study ($n = 50$) who underwent phacoemulsification. Density was graded into 0+, 1+, 2+, and 3+ (Nelson's classification of squamous metaplasia) and was reduced at 6 weeks (1.14 ± 0.88) compared to preoperatively (1.60 ± 0.93, $P < .001$) [13]. In 48 eyes, mean GCD calculated as the number of cells per square millimeter was reduced at day 1, 4 weeks, and 12 weeks ($p < 0.001$). Impression cytology demonstrated greater cell loss and conjunctival epithelium squamous metaplasia at day 1 compared to 1 and 3 months. Additionally, GCD decrease and surgery duration were correlated ($r^2 = .65$) [41]. A similar study reported metaplasia as more evident in the lower lid-covered area at 3 months, suggesting drops induction [42].

5.4 Cornea

Punctate keratopathy is reported to be predominantly in central cornea at day 1 in 40% and at day 7 in 32.7% in a study of 55 eyes with no prior DE. At 1 month, those still with keratopathy showed inferior quadrant predominance (21.8%) thought to be due to topical treatment persistence and lack of upper lid protection in this area [43].

Corneal sensitivity esthesiometer threshold in millimeters is significantly lower in both DE and no DE control groups at day 1 with 2.85 mm keratome incisions (55.1 ± 1.8,

51.2 ± 0.9, respectively) than preoperatively (58.4 ± 1.7, 55.9 ± 1.4, respectively). Sensitivity was more slowly recovered in the DE group than controls at 1 month (57.8 ± 1.5, 54.1 ± 1.2, respectively) and 2 months (58.1 ± 1.7, 56.1 ± 1.3, respectively) ($P < .05$, respectively) [35]. In a cohort with 2.8 mm incisions, center and temporal incision site sensitivity decreased at day 1 ($P = .021$, $P < .001$, respectively) but returned to preoperative levels at 1 month [41]. In 18 patients with 4.1 mm incisions, sensitivity did not return to baseline until 3 months [44]. More recently with confocal microscopy, a significant decrease in corneal vortical maximum length and average density ($P < .05$) has been observed, which lasted approximately 3 months.

In femtosecond laser-assisted cataract surgery (FLACS) with sustained vacuum eye coupling to the laser delivery system, worsened OSDI and Subjective Symptom Questionnaires were documented at day 1 and weeks 1, 4, and 12 (all $P < .001$) in 38 patients without DE previously. At 3 months, coincidental CFS score increases did not return to baseline ($P < .044$) despite ST-1 and TBUTs recovering to preoperative levels ($P = .062$ and $P = .306$, respectively) [45]. In a study comparing patients with no DE undergoing FLACS (n = 150 eyes) and conventional phacoemulsification (n = 150 eyes), OSDI and CFS scores in the FLACS group at day 1 and week 1 increased more significantly than in the conventional group. Scores did return to preoperative levels along with TBUT and ST-I values at 3 months (all $P > .05$) [46]. These findings are similar to and expand on those in an earlier study where there was comparatively significantly increased CFS at 1 month in the FLACS arm [47]. Another similar study, however, reported no significant changes to dry eye indices after FLACS and conventional phacoemulsification surgery [48].

Increased DE is noted after sutureless large incision manual cataract extraction [49], but no differences in DE have been noted between manual small-incision and conventional phacoemulsification [50–52]. No significant differences in DE have been noted between small-incision temporal corneal and superior corneoscleral tunnel approaches either [53].

6. Preoperative considerations

6.1 Risk factors

Few studies have investigated the local ocular surface and systemic conditions that cause DE and their impact post-surgery. With systemic disease, in a prospective, interventional case series comparing 174 diabetics without DE age-matched against 474 non-diabetics, diabetics had worse DE symptoms and TBUT after surgery. Incidence of DE was 17.1% in diabetics and 8.1% in non-diabetics at 7 days. In diabetics, DE incidence remained at 4.8% at 1 month but decreased to zero at 3 months. No DE was diagnosed in non-diabetics at 1 or 3 months [54]. In a small retrospective case series review of 15 patients, Sjogren's syndrome patients had poorer visual outcomes and increased complications postoperatively such as endophthalmitis and peripheral keratolysis as compared to dry eye patients without connective tissue disease [55].

A number of systemic factors are associated with persistent DE-like symptoms and DE Questionnaire-5 scores of ≥6 at 6 months, otherwise defined as persistent postsurgical pain (PSP) (**Table 1**) [56, 57]. In 119 patients (53 males; mean age 73 ± 6 years) PSP has been reported in 34% at 6 months. Frequency of severe PSP (DE Questionnaire-5 score ≥ 12) was 18% [56]. In a similar study, DE-like symptoms were reported in 32% (n = 27) of individuals 6 months postoperatively with 10% (n = 8)

Systemic association	OR	95% CI	P value
Antidepressants	3.17	1.31–7.68	.01[56]
Antihistamines	6.22	2.17–17.8	.0003[56]
Anti-insomnia medications	5.28	0.98–28.5	.047[56]
Anti-reflux medications	2.42	1.04–5.66	.04[56]
Anxiolytics	3.38	1.11–10.3	.03[56]
Autoimmune disorders	13.2	1.53–114	.007[56]
Female sex	2.68	1.20–6.00	.01[56]
Non-ocular chronic pain disorder (headache, migraine, low back pain, and fibromyalgia)	4.29 4.4	1.01–18.1 1.58–12.1	.06[56] .005[57]

Table 1.
Systemic associations with persistent postoperative dry eye symptoms.

having a DE Questionnaire-5 score ≥ 12 [57]. These patients had increased artificial tears usage ($P < .0001$), ocular pain ($P < .0001$), and neuropathic symptoms, including burning ($P < .001$), wind sensitivity ($P = .001$), and light sensitivity ($P < .0001$) [56]. These patients may be not be ideal multifocal IOL candidates.

One study by Min et al. examined the relationship between dry eye symptoms after cataract surgery and psychiatric status. They found higher OSDI scores at 3 months in the higher rather than lower depression and anxiety score groups. It was concluded that evaluation of patients' psychiatric status may help predict the severity of DE symptoms after cataract surgery and prepare for any post-operative DE management [58].

Regarding local conditions, 20 conjunctivochalasis patients were studied by our group. We recorded TMH as well as conjunctivochalasis fold height preoperatively using the Oculus Keratograph 5 M linear rule function and Meller and Tseng grading and observed unilateral clear corneal incision effects. At 1 month, there were increases in middle conjunctivochalasis fold height and absolute fold height to TMH ratio (0.35 ± 0.36 mm and 0.6 ± 0.7,) compared to baseline (0.2 ± 0.1 mm and 1.0 ± 0.9, $P = .029$ and .041, respectively). There was no significant difference in total and location-specific grade (both $P > .05$). Additionally, no statistically significant differences were noted in TBUT, osmolarity, Oxford staining, and ST-1 scores (Unpublished data). Sub-Tenon's blocks are associated with chemosis and subconjunctival hemorrhage [59]. We postulate that changes may relate to surgical influence, eyelid speculum, or local anesthesia but without significant DE impact at 4 weeks. Mimura et al. evaluated total change in severity after superior sclerocorneal incisions in 36 patients. Total grade increased significantly from 4.0 ± 1.9 at baseline to 4.8 ± 2.1 at 1 week ($P = .0048$) and decreased at 4 (4.3 ± 2.0) and 12 weeks (4.0 ± 1.9) [60].

6.2 Clinical diagnosis

A comprehensive algorithm that aids in preoperative DE diagnosis has been published [61]. More recently, the Ocular Surface Fraility Index, which incorporates 10 DE risk/contributing factors, has been published as a tool to predict the likelihood of DE symptoms at 1 and 3 months postoperatively [62]. Signs and symptoms of DE are, however, known to poorly correlate, and preoperative patients can often be asymptomatic even with advanced ocular surface disease (OSD) signs [61, 63]. It is also recognized that many, especially more elderly with significant cataracts, either do not have DE symptoms or feel the need to report them [61]. Nevertheless, symptom assessment is an integral part of preoperative work-up and is complementary to a focused examination as per the ASCRS Cornea Clinical Committee [63].

6.3 Investigations

Cataract surgery investigations aid prognostication of DE impact on outcomes. Biometry is influenced by DE such that it may be considered a DE investigation. Anterior corneal curvature is a major component of all IOL power calculation formulas [64]. An abnormal keratometry (K) reading can affect the accuracy of calculations and result in submaximal refractive results. Keratometry is sensitive to poor tear films as standard keratometers rely on good corneal reflection of mires [65]. Corneal power error differences of 1.0 diopter (D) result in approximately a 1.0 D error in postoperative refraction [66]. In 50 hyperosmolar subjects, higher average K reading variability ($P = .05$) and percentage of eyes with ≥1.0 D difference in corneal astigmatism ($P = .02$) was found as compared to 25 normals. Additionally, a higher percentage of eyes in the hyperosmolar group had IOL power differences of >0.5 D ($P = .02$). These findings signify that repeatable and reliable keratometry is necessary, especially with toric IOLs [64]. Lubricant viscosity can also adversely affect readings; thus, measurements should be made after 5 minutes [67]. Prior tear film stabilization is therefore crucial.

A systematic review of four studies has been conducted by Biela et al. that evaluated the effect of dry eye disease on biometric measurements before cataract surgery and postoperative refractive errors. The results unanimously indicated that refractive errors can be reduced by pre-treatment with substances such as topical Dexamethasone, Cyclosporin A, Loteprednol, and Lifitegrast [68]. A more recent study has been a single center, prospective, open-label study of 35 dry eyes prior to surgery, which has investigated baseline biometry and again after Rebamipide 2% suspension qid for 28 days. Improvement in anterior corneal tear film optical quality was demonstrated by significantly improved TBUT, superficial punctate keratopathy, and corneal higher order aberrations, which in turn increased accuracy of preoperative anterior corneal power measurements with significantly improved spherical equivalent refractive error prediction [69].

Corneal topography is able to confirm magnitude and axis of corneal astigmatism and is advocated prior to multifocal IOL insertion [65, 70]. Central corneal thickness measurements in one study comparing 34 DE patients and 28 healthy subjects have been shown to fluctuate in DE (repeated-measures analysis of variance, $P < .001$). Artificial tears improved measurement repeatability after 5 minutes [71]. In 33 female DE patients, central and mean mid-peripheral corneal thicknesses measured higher after artificial tears for 1 month ($P = .001$, $P = .02$) [72]. Not only are these responses to artificial tears useful in evaluating DE treatment but also examining the smoothness and spacing of reflected topography images for poor image quality can identify significant OSD [65, 72]. VERION™ keratometry allowing for intraoperative astigmatism axis digital marking is also affected with DE patients exhibiting more residual astigmatism if not lubricated 30 minutes prior [73].

6.4 Management

A number of recent studies have reported positive preoperative DE management results in optimization of postsurgical ocular surface health and refractive outcomes (**Table 2**), and it is advocated that OSD be treated aggressively preoperatively [65]. It is also suggested that surgery be delayed until OSD is managed to reduce postoperative complications, which are increased in DE disease [82]. Those with severe and/or progressive OSD are not good multifocal IOL candidates, but their use in selected, appropriately counseled, patients on a "case-by-case" basis has been ratified [65]. These patients, especially, would benefit from preoperative management. A comprehensive algorithm for management is published by Starr et al. [61].

Preoperative MGD management is reported in a prospective, randomized clinical trial of 120 moderate obstructive MGD patients. Sixty were assigned routine postoperative anti-inflammatory tobramycin 0.3/dexamethasone 0.1% drops. Thirty received preoperative warm moist compress (moist air and warmer mask, 40°C, 20 minutes) and massage (down or upward mild eyelid compression with finger, 10 minutes) as well as lid margin tobramycin 0.3%/dexamethasone 0.1% ointment bd and routine postoperative anti-inflammatory drops. The last 30 received enhanced postoperative anti-inflammatory treatment consisting of tobramycin 0.3%/dexamethasone 0.1% eye drops 6 times daily in the first week and qid in the second with frequency decreased by half every week the following 2 weeks. All received 0.1%

Study	Cohort	Design	Intervention	Results after surgery
Song et al. [74]	120 eyes	Single-center RCT	Moist air 40°C, warmer mask 20 minutes, massage, Oc Tobramycin 0.3%/ Dexamethasone 0.1% ointment bd pre-op + conventional post-op G Tobramycin 0.3/ Dexamethasone 0.1% and 0.1% Sodium hyaluronate versus Conventional post-op therapy	At 1 month, pre-op therapy arm presented higher noninvasive TBUTs, lower ocular symptoms scores, less lid margin abnormalities, and increased meibum quality and expressibility (All P < .001).
Favuzza et al. [75]	419 eyes	Retrospective multicenter review	1. Hydroxypropyl guar (HPG) and hyaluronic acid (HA) tds 1 week pre-op and 2 months post-op + conventional post-op G Nepafenac, Dexamethasone and Tobramycin 2. HPG and HA 2 months post-op + conventional post-op therapy 3. Conventional post-op therapy	In groups 1 and 2, SPEED scores were significantly lower than in group 3 in the whole 8-week post-op period. In group 1, SPEED scores were lower than in group 2, at 1 and 4 weeks after surgery (P < .001 and P = .021, respectively). TBUT in groups 1 and 2 was higher than in group 3 in the whole post-op period (P < .001). In group 1, TBUT was higher than in group 2, at 4 week (P = .016).
Fogagnolo et al. [76]	45 eyes	Multicenter, open label, RCT	Liposomal nanodispersion solution of omega 3, vitamins D and A tds (VisuoEvo, VISUfarma, Netherlands) 2 weeks pre-op to 2 weeks post-op + conventional post-op therapy of G Dexamethasone and Ofloxacin versus Conventional post-op therapy	At 1- and 2-weeks, pre-op therapy arm TBUT was higher than baseline (P < .01). At 1- and 2-weeks, pre-op therapy arm OSDI was lower than baseline (P < .027). Post-op CFS showed a much higher proportion of patients with optimal ocular surface protection in the VisuEvo group. The two groups did not show any significant differences in osmometry and ST-1.

Study	Cohort	Design	Intervention	Results after surgery
Donnenfeld et al. [77]	28 eyes	Multicenter contralaterally controlled double-masked trial	Cyclosporine 0.05% bd 1 month pre-op to 2 months post-op in 1 eye + conventional post-op therapy of Gatifloxacin, Ketorolac, and Prednisolone qid versus Artificial tear containing polyethylene glycol (Systane Free) in the other eye + conventional therapy	At 2 months post-op, the cyclosporine group had lower mean uncorrected and corrected distance visual acuity and CFS than the artificial tear group (P = .045, P = .005 and P = .034) Treatment with cyclosporine Significantly more patients preferred the eye treated with cyclosporine 0.05% to the eye treated with artificial tears (57.1% versus 14.3%; P = .007).
Ganesh et al. [78]	67 eyes	Single-center RCT	1. Cyclosporine 0.05% bd (Cyclotears, Entod pharmaceuticals, India) and 1% Carboxymethyl Cellulose (CMC) qid 2 weeks pre-op and 3 months post-op + conventional post-op Pred Forte, Nepafenac and Moxifloxacin 2. CMC qid + conventional therapy 3. Conventional post-op therapy	Group 1 showed improved osmolarity, TBUT, and ST-1 at 3 months compared to pre-op and week 1 but not groups 2 and 3 (All P < .001).
Shokoohi-Rad et al. [79]	62 eyes	Single-center triple-blind RCT	1. Bethamethasone 0.1% qid 4 days pre-op + conventional post-op therapy of Betamethasone 0.1% for 4 weeks and Levofloxacin 2. Normal saline 0.9% qid 4 days pre-op + conventional post-op therapy	OSDI and meniscometry were not affected by the interaction between time and Betamethasone (P = .192 and P = .578, respectively).
Lee et al. [80]	64 eyes	Retrospective, compartive, observational case series	1. Diquafosol 3% 6 times a day 1 week pre-op and 3 months post-op + conventional therapy of Gatifloxacin qid and Pred Forte qid for 4 weeks 2. Conventional post-op therapy	In group I, TBUT, OSDI and OSS showed improvement at one- and three-months post-op (P = .002 for BUT at 1 and 3 months, P = .023 and P = .049 for OSDI at 1 month and 3 months and P = .001 and P = .026 for OSS at 1 and 3 months) but not group 2. In both groups, ST-I decreased at 3 months post-op (P = .011, group I and P = .034, group 2), compared to baseline. No differences between the groups for corneal aberration.
Ge et al. [81]	60 eyes	Prospective observational study	M22 Optimal Pulsed Technology pre-op and at 1- and 2-months post-op + conventional post-op drops therapy of Levofloxacin and cortisone	Significant improvements in TBUT, CFS, TMH and MGYSS at 3 months post-op compared to baseline (All P < .05)

Table 2.
Clinical trials in the treatment of dry eye pre-cataract surgery.

sodium hyaluronate qid for 1 month. At 1 month, MGD showed aggravated status in Cohorts I and III but resolved by 3 months. At 1 month, Cohorts II and III presented higher noninvasive TBUTs, lower ocular symptoms scores, less lid margin abnormalities, and increased meibum quality and expressibility (Cohort II vs. I: all $P < .001$, respectively; Cohort III vs. I: $P = .011$, $P = .024$, $P = .046$, $P = .045$, and $P = .012$, respectively). Additionally, Cohort II had better lid margins and meibum quality and expressibility than Cohort III at 1 month ($P = .031$, $P = .026$, and $P < .001$, respectively). At 3 months, Cohort II presented higher noninvasive TBUTs than Cohorts I and III ($P < .001$ and $P = .001$, respectively) [74].

Cataract surgery outcomes in graft-versus-host disease (GVHD) have been studied with respect to DE as it is the most common ocular occurrence of this condition [83]. Along with DE, cataracts are a common cause of visual loss in GVHD [84]. Four studies, cumulatively examining 128 eyes of GVHD cataract surgery patients, demonstrated that maximal preoperative DE and other ocular surface therapy can gain significant mean visual acuity improvements. Local therapies included preservative free lubricants, 10% acetylcysteine and autologous serum eye drops, topical corticosteroids, cyclosporine-A and 0.1% tacrolimus in ointment form, bandage contact lens with topical antibiotics, scleral lenses, punctal occlusion, and moisture chamber goggles. Systemic therapies included omega-3-dietary supplements, steroids, cyclosporine-A, mycophenolate, and oral pilocarpine and cessation of systemic medications that could reduce tear production [85–88]. One study measured DE disease severity and OSDI pre- and post-surgery and observed a nonsignificant trend toward worsening [86]. Within 2 weeks, Balaram et al. noted worsening of OSD in 2 patients with one proceeding to corneal thinning. Both cases neglected restarting topical lubricants [85]. At 4 weeks, recurrence of ocular surface inflammation occurred in 7 eyes with cessation of topical and systemic immunosuppressive therapy in one study [85], while in another, 1 sterile corneal ulcer and 1 infected ulcer with perforations were reported in 2 severely DE patients along with band keratopathy [86]. Late corneal melts occurred in 2 patients some months later [88]. Penn and Soong reported no ocular surface complications [87].

Stevens-Johnson syndrome (SJS) patients undergoing cataract surgery are also reported to achieve good visual good outcomes following aggressive ocular surface stabilization preoperatively. Local therapeutic modalities are similar to those in GVHD but also include amniotic membrane grafting, symblepharon release, lash epilation/electrolysis, lid margin mucous membrane grafting, tarsorrhaphy, entropion correction, MGD management, and dacryocystectomy [89, 90]. Oral therapies include corticosteroids and methotrexate [90]. In 40 chronic SJS sequelae eyes, median preoperative LogMAR best-corrected visual acuity (BCVA) was 1.61 (IQR, 0.80 to 2.78). Median BCVA increased to 0.60 (IQR, 0.30 to 1.48, $P < .0001$). The ocular surface remained stable in 35 eyes (87.5%), but breakdown occurred in four (10%). Another study of 3 SJS eyes also reported BCVA gain and maintenance of ocular surface integrity [89].

7. Intraoperative considerations

Topical anesthesia can generate shorter admissions and lower cost phacoemulsification [91]. Tetracaine 0.5% absorption and duration is slow and short acting, necessitating repeated administration with corneal epithelial damage toxicity risk including punctate keratopathy and persistent epithelial defects. Lidocaine gel 2% is shown to allow significantly less administration while being more effective in relieving pain compared to tetracaine 0.5% due to greater concentration and longer epithelial contact time [92].

Eyelid speculums may cause MGD through lid dysfunction and inadequate meibum release [35]. A significant reduction in both levator function and marginal reflex distance 1 at 1, 30, and 90 days, which normalizes at 180 days, is reported [93]. Aspirating speculums also increase conjunctival staining at day 1 ($P = .001$), conjunctivochalasis grades at day 1 and 7 ($P < .001$), and OSDI at day 7 ($P = .011$) and reduce TBUT at days 1 and 7 ($P < .001$), perhaps through conjunctival aspiration through the suction holes. In comparison, non-aspirating speculums showed only TBUT and conjunctivochalasis grades significance at day 1 ($P < 0.001$). All parameters returned to baseline in both groups at 1 month [94].

Povidone-iodine antiseptic preparations cause DE. Epithelial cell cytotoxicity is linked to low iodine pH, osmolarity, and presence of lauromacrogol, which is a surfactant. Repeated ocular surface irrigation may also impact GCD and tear-film stability [95]. Ophthalmic viscosurgical devices (OVDs) may reduce cataract surgery trauma caused by ocular surface inflammatory mediator release [96, 97]. Intraoperative use of hydroxypropyl methocellulose (HPMC) 2% has been shown to significantly reduce balanced saline solution (BSS) application frequency intraoperatively in a HPMC group of 30 eyes compared to 30 eyes irrigated only with BSS ($p = 0.001$). Incidence of DE was significantly reduced in the HPMC group in both senile and diabetic patients. Subjective symptom scores were higher in the BSS group at day 1 ($P = .003$) and day 3 ($P = .043$). Noninvasive TBUTs were higher in the HPMC group at days 1 and 3 ($P = .012$ and $P = .024$, respectively). Values for TBUT did not significantly change postoperatively in the HPMC group, while they were significantly lower in the BSS group [98]. A similar study of 149 male eyes randomly assigned to receive HPMC 2% or BSS demonstrated that week 1 ST-1 values in the HPMC group were higher than those in the BSS group ($P = .019$). Patients with DE before surgery had 1-month post-op ST-1 values in the HPMC group higher than in the BSS group ($P = .037$). Additionally, in preoperative DE patients with surgical times longer than median, patients' CFS in the HPMC group was superior to that of the BSS group ($P = .032$) [96]. A polysaccharide gel of hydroxypropyl methylcellulose, xanthan gum, and carrageenan (eyeDRO; Alchimia, Italy) on the cornea in 28 eyes achieved return of TBUTs to preoperative levels by day 5 as compared to day 30 in the BSS group of 26 patients. Concordantly, OSDI returned to preoperative values after 15 days in the gel group and 30 days in the BSS group [99]. Reductions in TBUT, corneal ocular staining score, and OSDI are also reported with DisCoVisc (Alcon Laboratories, Fort Worth, TX, USA) in 13 patients (All $P < .01$) as compared to a BSS group 1 week postoperatively [100].

Corneal incisions reduce corneal sensitivity, which gradually recovers [35, 41, 44]. On corneal wounding, nerves are excited and local inflammation is produced through neuropeptide release. They also become sensitized by local inflammatory mediators and demonstrate spontaneous activity and enhanced responses to new stimuli generating spontaneous pain and hyperalgesia. Injured nerves also regenerate and form microneuromas that exhibit abnormal responsiveness and spontaneous discharges, which may also lead to spontaneous pain, DE sensations, and other dysesthesias [101]. Corneal innervation or lacrimal functional unit feedback disruption can lower tear production and blink rate with resultant tear film instability [11, 102]. Sufficient regeneration, however, results in DE transience postoperatively [13, 103]. Today's microincisions are assumed to generate less reduction in corneal sensitivity [35, 101].

Given that the large long ciliary nerves enter the limbus predominantly at 9 and 3 o'clock and corneal sensation is significantly greater at the temporal and nasal limbus, Cho et al. examined corneal incision location and impact on DE indices [104, 105]. No significant differences were found between superiorly versus temporally placed incisions with respect to TBUT, DE symptoms, ST-1, and TMH in both DE and non-DE groups [104].

Surgery duration affects the ocular surface commencing from operating microscope usage. Correlation of DE signs and symptoms have been shown to inversely correlate with microscope light exposure duration up until week 6 in a prospective study of 50 eyes with no DE signs or symptoms. These include means of OSDI ($P < .015$), ST-1 ($P < .003$), TBUT ($P < .011$), and CFS grades ($P < .003$) [13]. In another prospective study of 28 eyes with preoperative DE and 70 without preoperative DE, significant correlations were detected in the DE group between light exposure time and TBUT and DE symptoms at day 1 but not from day 3 onward. In the non-DE group, significant correlations were noted between light exposure time and DE symptoms at 1, 3, and 10 days and 2 months and in TBUT at 2 months [104]. A prospective observational study of 100 eyes also observed correlations of DE test values with light exposure time, but they were not significant [106].

Prolonged operating can increase cumulative dispersed energy with correlations found between DE test values and phacoemulsification energy used. In Kohli et al.'s study, a correlation was found between increased effective phacoemulsification time, which was used as a measure of phacoemulsification energy and reductions in OSDI ($P < .020$), Schirmer's I values ($P < .002$), TBUT ($P < .001$), and CFS grades ($P < .001$) up until 6 weeks [13]. Sahu et al. recorded cumulative dissipated energy, and although this was negatively correlated with ST-1, TBUT, and TMH, this was not statistically significant [106]. No correlations are also reported between energy and TBUT, DE symptoms, ST-1, and TMH in both DE and non-DE cohorts [104].

Eyedrops containing active agents/preservatives can adversely affect epithelium [95]. Intraoperative anterior chamber intracameral dexamethasone drug-delivery suspension (Dexycu; Icon Bioscience Inc., Newark, CA) was evaluated in a prospective, randomized 2:1, open-label, multicenter Phase III that may minimize postoperative drops use. Dexycu 517 μg 5 μL was administered to 126 patients through cannula insertion into the ciliary sulcus after IOL placement, and 55 patients received prednisolone 0.1% drops (1 drop 4 times daily for 3 weeks). At day 8, 51.6% of Dexycu eyes and 50.9% of prednisolone eyes had anterior chamber cell clearing; more than 98% had clearing at 90 days. There was no significant difference in endothelial cell density between groups. Steroid-related intraocular pressure rise was the most common adverse event (11.1%), then iritis (6.3%). In those receiving Dexycu, 68.7% strongly agreed that no eyedrop usage was very convenient, while 39.2% of those using prednisolone strongly agreed that they would prefer dropless therapy [107]. A similar Phase III study comparing 5 μl injections of 342 or 517 μg Dexycu showed comparable efficacy between both groups, with significantly increased anterior chamber cell and flare clearing compared to placebo [108].

A bandage contact lens (PureVision; Bausch & Lomb Inc., Rochester, NY) at surgery completion in 30 patients with mild MGD was shown on 1 week removal to improve OSDI, subjective evaluation scores, TBUT and CFS compared to 30 MGD controls without contact lens, especially on days 7 and 14 ($P < .001$, $P < .001$; $P = .031$, $P = .009$; $P = .021$, $P = .028$; and $P = .03$, $P = .032$, respectively). At days 30 and 90, there were no significant differences between groups and in BCVA or Schirmer values [109].

8. Postoperative considerations

A number of DE treatments have been trialed with varying measures of success (**Table 3**). There appears to be scope for further trials with the newer

Study	Cohort	Design	Intervention	Results after surgery
Tyson et al. [110]	438 eyes	Multicenter Phase III RCT	Intracanalicular 0.4 mg Dexamethasone insert (Dextenza; Ocular Therapeutix, Bedford, MA) versus Placebo	At day 14, absence of anterior chamber cells in insert arm greater than placebo (52.3% versus 31%; $P < .0001$). At day 8, absence of ocular pain in insert arm greater than placebo (79.6% versus 61.3%; $P < .0001$). Insert arm showed no increase compared with placebo in incidence of all adverse events or ocular adverse events.
Walters et al. [111]	60 eyes	Multicenter double-masked RCT	Intracanalicular 0.4 mg Dexamethasone suspended in a dried polyethylene glycol hydrogel insert. The hydrogel is conjugated with fluorescein to assist visualization versus Placebo	At day 8 20.7% of patients in insert arm with absence of anterior chamber cells compared with 10.0% in placebo group ($P \leq .1495$). At day 8, absence of ocular pain in insert arm greater than placebo (79.3% versus 30.0%; $p < .0001$) and at all other timepoint versts through 30 days post-op ($P < .0002$). At several timepoints through 30 days, absence of anterior chamber cells, anterior chamber flare, and pain was greater in insert arm than placebo ($P \leq .0251$).
Jee et al. [112]	80 eyes	Single-center RCT	Fluorometholone 0.1% PF qid, Sodium hyaluronate PF 0.1% qid + Gatifloxacin 0.3% qid for 4 weeks then all tds for 4 weeks versus Preserved Fluorometholone 0.1% (Ocumetholone), Preserved Sodium hyaluronate 0.1% (Lacure) + Gatifloxacin 0.3% on same schedule	At 2 months, OSDI, TBUT, ST-I, CFS, impression cytology, and GCD were better in Group 1 than in Group 2 (All $P < .05$). At 2 months, interleukin-1b and tumor necrosis factor-a concentrations were less in the tears of Group 1 than in the tears of Group 2, and catalase and superoxide dismutase 2 fluorescence intensities were greater in the tears of Group 1 than in the tears of Group 2 (All $P < .05$).
Chung et al. [113]	32 dry eyes	Single-center RCT	Cyclosporine 0.05% bd 1 week post-op (Restasis; Allergan Inc., Irvine, CA) for 3 months versus Normal saline 0.9% bd 1 week post-op for 3 months	At 3 months, greater improvement in ST-I in Cyclosporine arm compared with control ($P = .02$). At 1 month, improvement in TBUT with Cyclosporine and increases seen at 2 and 3 months ($P = .04$, $P < .01$, respectively). No significant increases seen in control group at any timepoint. At 3 months, Cyclosporine arm showed improvement for each OSDI score ($P < .01$, $P = .01$, $P = .02$, respectively).
Kudyar et al. [114]	69 dry eyes	Prospective randomized open-label study	Cyclosporine 0.1% bd + CMC 0.5% tds 1-week post-op for 8 weeks versus CMC 0.5% tds 1-week post-op for 8 weeks	Treatment in both groups cyclosporine 0.1% + artificial tears 0.5% and artificial tears 0.5% led to improvement in OSDI at 4 and 8 weeks ($P < .0001$) Difference between the mean values of the two groups was significant both at 4 ($P < .0001$) and 8 weeks ($P < .0001$)

Study	Cohort	Design	Intervention	Results after surgery
Baek et al. [115]	68 dry eyes	Prospective RCT	Diquafosol 3% qid 1-week post-op for 8 weeks versus Normal saline 0.9% qid 1-week post-op for 8 weeks	At 8 weeks, TBUT, and CFS improved in Diquafosol arm (P < .01, P < .01) and were better than normal saline (P < .01, P < .01). ST-1 did not improve (P = .26). All symptom questionnaire scores improved in eyes treated with 3.0% Diquafosol (All P < .01).
Cui et al. [116]	94 dry eyes	Prospective open-label RCT	Diquafosol 3% (Diquas; Santen Pharmaceutical Co, Ltd., Osaka, Japan) qid for 12 weeks versus Sodium hyaluronate (SH) 0.1% (Kynex, Alcon) qid for 12 weeks.	Conjunctival squamous metaplasia grade was lower at 12 weeks, and GCD was higher at 4 and 12 weeks in the Cyclosporine group than in the hyaluronate group (P < .05). Cyclosporine group showed lower OSDI scores at 4 and 12 weeks; longer TBUT at 1, 4, and 12 weeks; lower keratoepitheliopathy scores at 1 and 12 weeks; and lower spherical aberrations at 4 weeks after surgery (P < .05).
Miyake et al. [117]	154 dry eyes	Open-label RCT	Diquafosol 3% 6 times a day 4 weeks post-op for 4 weeks versus Artificial tears 6 times a day 4 weeks post-op for 4 weeks	TBUT was prolonged in the DQS group (*P* = 0.015), but not in the AT group. Fluorescein staining score was significantly improved in both groups (*P*,0.001).
Park et al. [118]	130 dry eyes	Prospective RCT	Diquafosol 3% 6 times a day (Diquas®; Santen Pharmaceutical Co, Ltd., Osaka, Japan) for 12 weeks post-op versus Sodium hyaluronate 0.1% 6 times a day for 12 weeks post-op	Diquafosol showed superior TBUT (P < .001), CFS (P < .045), and conjunctival staining (P < .001) compared to Sodium hyaluronate throughout the study period. TBUT (P < .001) and change in HOAs (P < .018) recovered more quickly in the Diquafosol group.
Jun et al. [119]	117 dry eyes	Prospective RCT	1. Diquafosol 3% PF* 6 times a day 2. Diquafosol 3% with preservatives^ 6 times a day 3. Sodium hyaluronate 0.15% PF 6 times a day (All groups for 12 weeks) (*Diquas-S; ^Diquas; Santen Pharmaceutical Co, Ltd., Osaka, Japan)	Group 1 improved TBUT, OSDI, CFS scores, lid margin abnormality, and meibum quality over time. Groups 1 and 2 had superior TBUT, MGD grade, and MGE throughout the study than Group 3 (All P < .001). Group 1 Meibum quality was better than Group 2 at 3 months (P < .001).
Lee et al. [120]	40 dry eyes	Single-center RCT	Diquafosol 3% 6 times a day 1-week post-op to 3 months post-op versus Cyclosporine A 0.05% bd 1-week post-op to 3 months post-op	Diquafosol showed higher TBUT outcomes than Cyclosporine A at 1 (P < 0.001) at 3 months (P = .001). Cyclosporine A showed more decreased vertical coma and total HOAs than Diquafosol at 3 months (Both P < .01).

Study	Cohort	Design	Intervention	Results after surgery
Inoue et al. [121]	59 dry eyes	Post-hoc analysis of RCT	Diquafosol 3% 6 times a day (Diquas®; Santen Pharmaceutical Co, Ltd., Osaka, Japan) 4 weeks post-op for 4 weeks versus Artificial tears 6 times a day (Mytear®; Senju Pharmaceutical Co., Ltd., Osaka, Japan) 4 weeks post-op for 4 weeks	Diquafosol increase in TBUT was greater than artificial tears at 8 weeks (P = .014). Diquafosol showed lower HOA fluctuations and changes than artificial tears at 8 weeks (Both, P = .004).
Kato et al. [122]	80 eyes	Two-center RCT	1. Diclofenac 0.1% PF tds 2. Rebamipide 2%* qid + Diclofenac 0.1% PF tds 3. Betamethasone 0.1% PF tds 4. Rebamipide 2% qid + Betamethasone 0.1% PF tds (*Mucosta; Otsuka Pharmaceutical Co, Ltd., Tokyo, Japan)	Group 1 mean (± SD) GCD before surgery was 257.0 ± 188.7 cells/mm^2, and it decreased significantly to 86.5 ± 76.7 cells/mm^2 at 1 month (P = .002). Groups 2, 3, and 4 showed no significant differences in GCD at 1 month.
Yao et al. [123]	180 eyes	Multi-center RCT	Carboxymethylcellulose sodium (CMC) 1% qid (Refresh Liquigel; Allergan, Inc., Irvine, CA) + Conventional therapy of Prednisolone acetate 1% qid and Levofloxacin 0.5% qid versus Conventional therapy	CMC group had increased TBUT compared with control at day 7 (P = .0475) and day 30 (P = .0258). CMC group with a pre-surgical diagnosis of DE had increased TBUT (P < .001 at both day 7 and 30). Control group with no prior diagnosis of DE had decreased TBUT (P < .02 at both day 7 and 30).
Sanchez et al.	48 eyes	Single-center RCT	HP-Guar (Systane UD, Alcon Cusí, Spain) qid post-op for 1 month + conventional therapy of G Tobramycin and G Dexamethasone qid tapering over 4 weeks versus Conventional therapy	At 4 weeks, HP-Guar group showed better TBUT (P < .0004), OSDI (P < .0002), ocular symptoms (P < .0004), vision-related function (P < .0002) and reduced expression of CD3 (P < .011), and HLA-DR (P < .0002) inflammatory markers.
Mencucci et al. [124]	282 eyes	Multicenter RCT	Sodium hyaluronate 0.1% qid and CMC 0.5% qid post-op for 5 weeks + conventional therapy of 4 weeks of tapering Tobramycin 0.3% and dexamethasone acetate 0.1% versus Conventional therapy	At 5 weeks, TBUT was higher in the study group than in controls (P < .0003). At 5 weeks, dry-eye symptoms improved in the study group compared with controls (P < .001). At 5 weeks, CFS was significantly reduced in the study group compared with controls (P < .002 versus P < .05, respectively).

Study	Cohort	Design	Intervention	Results after surgery
Caretti et al. [125]	60 dry eyes	Single-center Randomized case–control study	Carbomer sodium hyaluronate trehalose eye drops bd (Thealoz Gel®, Thea Laboratoires, Clermont-Ferrand, France) + Conventional therapy of topical steroid-antibiotic and NSAID versus Sodium hyaluronate bd (Hydrabak®, Thea Laboratoires, Clermont-Ferrand, France) + Conventional therapy	Trehalose group showed a significantly greater TBUT increase compared to hyaluronate group at day 30 ($P < .001$). Trehalose group showed a significantly greater improvement in OSDI compared to hyaluronate group at day 30 ($P < .001$).
Jee et al. [112]	80 dry eyes	2 groups RCT	Sodium hyaluronate 0.1% preservative-free (Tearin free) and Fluorometholone 0.1% eyedrops preservative-free (Humeron) versus Sodium hyaluronate 0.1% with preservatives (Lacure) and Fluorometholone 0.1% eyedrops with preservatives (Ocumetholone) Both groups at qid for the 1st month and then bd for the 2nd month	At 2 months, OSDI, TBUT, ST-1, CFS score, impression cytology findings, and goblet cell count were significantly better in Group 1 than in Group 2 ($P < .05$). At 2 months, IL-1beta and TNF-alpha concentrations were significantly less in Group 1 patient tears than in Group 2 patient tears, and catalase and superoxide dismutase 2 fluorescence intensities were significantly greater in Group 1 patient tears than in Group 2 ($P < .05$).
Mohamma-dpour et al. [126]	62 dry eyes	Triple-blinded RCT	Treatment group of artificial tears (Artelac; Bausch & Lomb, Rochester, NY, USA), topical steroid (betamethasone 1%) drops and eye shampoos (constituents: Rewopol, Rewoteric, HEC, PEG-40 hydrogenated castor oil) containing tea tree oil 4 weeks after surgery versus Control group of artificial tears, topical steroids, and eye shampoos without tea tree oil 4 weeks after surgery	Tear breakup time, osmolarity, and OSDI scores in the treatment group were significantly better than those in the control group ($P < .05$) at 8 weeks. *Demodex* decreased only in the treatment group after treatment ($P < .001$) at 8 weeks. There was no significant difference between the two groups in the pre- and post-ST test results ($P > .05$) at 8 weeks.
Mohamma-dpour et al. [127]	61 dry eyes	Triple-blinded RCT	Omega-3 dietary supplement every 8 hours (1000 mg Advanced® Canada, each capsule containing 180 mg EPA and 120 mg DHA) + Conventional therapy of artificial tears qid (Artelac; Dr. Gerhard Mann Chem-pharm Fabrik GmbH, Berlin, Germany) versus Conventional therapy only control	No significant difference between control and treatment groups in mean postoperative time at trial start (1.61 ± 1.60 and 1.57 ± 1.57 years, respectively, $P > .930$). Omega-3 improvement in OSDI was higher than control at 1 month, ($P = .026$). Omega-3 increased TBUT more than control at 1 month ($P = .038$). Mean pre-treatment tear film osmolarity in the treatment group was 315.40 ± 17.06 (range: 279–340), which improved to 296.90 ± 14.39 (range: 260–310) at 1 month ($P < .001$). Mean tear film osmolarity in the control group improved insignificantly at 1 month.

Study	Cohort	Design	Intervention	Results after surgery
Park et al. [128]	66 dry eyes 1 month after surgery	Prospective comparative cohort study	Re-esterified triglyceride form of Omega-3, 2 tablets bd (total = 1680 mg EPA/506 mg DHA) for 8 weeks (PRN Dry Eye Omega Benefits softgels; PRN Physician Recommended Nutriceuticals, Plymouth Meeting, Pennsylvania, USA) + lubricant qid versus Lubricant qid	OSS was lower in the omega-3 group than in the control group ($P < .05$). There was an improvement of OSDI and DEQ in the omega-3 group (Both $P < .05$). The ratio of increasing MMP-9 level in the omega-3 group was lower than that in the control group ($P = .027$).
Son et al. [129]	40 dry eyes	Single-center open-label CT	100% perfluorohexyloctane qid (EvoTears; URSAPHARM, GmbH) + Conventional therapy of (Isopto Max eye drops and Isopto Max eye ointment; Novartis Pharma GmbH)	At 5 weeks, mean TBUT value (13.5 ± 6.7 s) increased ($P < .001$) compared to preoperatively (6.5 ± 1.6 s) At 5 weeks, mean total CFS score (2.36 ± 2.03) improved ($P < .004$) compared to preoperatively (3.53 ± 2.00)
Devendra et al. [130]	64 eyes	Single-center RCT	Oral lactoferrin 350 gm versus Without oral lactroferrin control	At day 60, TBUT of control group was 7.86 (±0.86) seconds as compared to 13.9(± 0.99) seconds in the lactoferrin group. At day 60, ST-1 values also showed a statistically significant difference between the two groups - 15.86 (± 5.83) seconds in the control group versus 30.9 (± 1.66) in the lactoferrin group.

RCT = randomized control trial; ST-I = Schirmer's Test I; TBUT = tear breakup time; OSDI = Ocular Surface Disease Index; OSS = Oxford corneal staining score; DEQ = Dry Eye Questionnaire; CFS = corneal fluorescein staining; MGD = Meibomian gland dysfunction; MGE = Meibomian gland expression; HOA = higher order aberrations; SD = standard deviation; GCD = goblet cell density; CMC = carboxymethylcellulose sodium; DE = dry eye.

Table 3.
Clinical trials in the treatment of dry eye post-cataract surgery.

anti-inflammatories appearing on the market potentially in severe DE cataract patients. More cost-effective combination therapies could also be trialed across the spectrum.

9. Conclusions

Successful cataract surgery is a rewarding experience, but patients and surgeons may be dissatisfied when DE predominates recovery. Patients can be reassured that ocular surface normalization usually occurs within 3 months, but persistent DE is a risk for a clinically significant minority. This can detract from vision quality and manifest as persistent surgical pain. It may be especially problematic in multifocal IOL patients where premium prices have been paid and no highly expected quality of life improvement has been forthcoming. An understanding of the pre-, intra-, and postoperative factors that influence the refractive results in OSD allows both clinicians and patients to have more reasonable expectations and tailored strategies to achieve desired outcomes. This review of the English literature sets the scene for more holistic care and research of cataract surgery patients with DE as more advances are made available to us in the ever-evolving premium lens and DE landscapes.

Author details

Kenneth Gek-Jin Ooi*, King Fai Calvin Leung, Jessica Xiong, Pauline Khoo and Stephanie Louise Watson
Discipline of Ophthalmology, Sydney Medical School, Save Sight Institute, The University of Sydney, Sydney, Australia

*Address all correspondence to: kenneth.ooi@sydney.edu.au

References

[1] Vinson JA. Oxidative stress in cataracts. Pathophysiology. 2006;**13**(3):151-162

[2] Seen S, Tong L. Dry eye disease and oxidative stress. Acta Ophthalmologica. 2018;**96**(4):e412-e420

[3] Bradley JL et al. Dry eye disease ranking among common reasons for seeking eye care in a large US claims database. Clinical Ophthalmology. 2019;**13**:225-232

[4] Liu Y-C et al. Cataracts. The Lancet. 2017;**390**(10094):600-612

[5] Lee C, Afshari N. The global state of cataract blindness. Current Opinion in Ophthalmology. 2017;**28**(1):98-103

[6] Foreman KJ et al. Forecasting life expectancy, years of life lost, and all-cause and cause-specific mortality for 250 causes of death: Reference and alternative scenarios for 2016-40 for 195 countries and territories. The Lancet. 2018;**392**(10159):2052-2090

[7] Craig JP et al. TFOS DEWS II definition and classification report. The Ocular Surface. 2017;**15**(3):276-283

[8] Wolffsohn JS et al. TFOS DEWS II diagnostic methodology report. The Ocular Surface. 2017;**15**(3):539-574

[9] Messmer EM. The pathophysiology, diagnosis, and treatment of dry eye disease. Deutsches Arzteblatt International. 2015;**112**(5):71-82

[10] Donthineni PR, Das AV, Shanbhag SS, Basu S. Cataract surgery in dry eye disease: Visual outcomes and complications. Frontiers in Medicine (Lausanne). 7 Oct 2020;7:575834

[11] Kasetsuwan N et al. Incidence and pattern of dry eye after cataract surgery. PLoS One. 2013;**8**(11):e78657-e78657

[12] Alio JL et al. Multifocal intraocular lenses: An overview. Survey of Ophthalmology. 2017;**62**(5):611-634

[13] Kohli P et al. Changes in ocular surface status after phacoemulsification in patients with senile cataract. International Ophthalmology. 2019;**39**(6):1345-1353

[14] Galor A et al. Intraocular lens exchange surgery in dissatisfied patients with refractive intraocular lenses. Journal of Cataract & Refractive Surgery. 2009;**35**(10):1706-1710

[15] Montés-Micó R et al. Visual performance with multifocal intraocular lenses: Mesopic contrast sensitivity under distance and near conditions. Ophthalmology. 2004;**111**(1):85-96

[16] Leyland M, Pringle E. Multifocal versus monofocal intraocular lenses after cataract extraction. Cochrane Database of Systematic Reviews. 18 Oct 2006;(4):CD003169

[17] de Vries NE et al. Intraocular straylight after implantation of the multifocal AcrySof ReSTOR SA60D3 diffractive intraocular lens. Journal of Cataract & Refractive Surgery. 2008;**34**(6):957-962

[18] Szczotka-Flynn LB et al. Impact of dry eye on visual acuity and contrast sensitivity: Dry eye assessment and management study. Optometry and Vision Science: Official Publication of the American Academy of Optometry. 2019;**96**(6):387-396

[19] Woodward MA, Randleman JB, Stulting RD. Dissatisfaction after

multifocal intraocular lens implantation. Journal of Cataract and Refractive Surgery. 2009;**35**(6):992-997

[20] Gibbons A et al. Causes and correction of dissatisfaction after implantation of presbyopia-correcting intraocular lenses. Clinical Ophthalmology. 2016;**10**:1965-1970

[21] Ahn JM et al. Prevalence of and risk factors associated with dry eye: The Korea National Health and nutrition examination survey 2010-2011. American Journal of Ophthalmology. 2014;**158**(6):1205-1214.e7

[22] Moss SE, Klein R, Klein BEK. Prevalance of and risk factors for dry eye syndrome. Archives of Ophthalmology. 2000;**118**(9):1264-1268

[23] Siffel C et al. Burden of dry eye disease in Germany: A retrospective observational study using German claims data. Acta Ophthalmologica. 2020;**98**(4):e504-e512

[24] Vehof J, Snieder H, Jansonius N, Hammond CJ. Prevalence and risk factors of dry eye in 79,866 participants of the population-based lifelines cohort study in the Netherlands. Ocular Surface. Jan 2021;**19**:83-93

[25] Xue W et al. Long-term impact of dry eye symptoms on vision-related quality of life after phacoemulsification surgery. International Ophthalmology. 2019;**39**(2):419-429

[26] Trattler WB et al. The prospective health assessment of cataract Patients' ocular surface (PHACO) study: The effect of dry eye. Clinical Ophthalmology (Auckland, N.Z.). 2017;**11**:1423-1430

[27] Szakáts I et al. Dry eye symptoms, patient-reported visual functioning, and health anxiety influencing patient satisfaction after cataract surgery. Current Eye Research. 2017;**42**(6):832-836

[28] Ishrat S, Nema N, Chandravanshi SCL. Incidence and pattern of dry eye after cataract surgery. Saudi Journal of Ophthalmology : Official Journal of the Saudi Ophthalmological Society. 2019;**33**(1):34-40

[29] Hanyuda A et al. Discrepancies in persistent dry eye signs and symptoms in bilateral Pseudophakic patients. Journal of Clinical Medicine. 2019;**8**(2):211

[30] Cetinkaya S et al. The course of dry eye after phacoemulsification surgery. BMC Ophthalmology. 2015;**15**:68-68

[31] El Ameen A et al. Influence of cataract surgery on Meibomian gland dysfunction. Journal Français d'Ophtalmologie. 2018;**41**(5):e173-e180

[32] Han KE et al. Evaluation of dry eye and Meibomian gland dysfunction after cataract surgery. American Journal of Ophthalmology. 2014;**157**(6):1144-1150.e1

[33] Cung LX, Nga NTT, Nga DM, Hiep NX, Pham DT. Cataract surgery destabilises temporary the tear film of the ocular surface. Klinische Monatsblatter fur Augenheilkunde. Mar 2021;**238**(3):282-287

[34] Shimabukuro M et al. Effects of cataract surgery on symptoms and findings of dry eye in subjects with and without preexisting dry eye. Japanese Journal of Ophthalmology. 2020;**64**(4):429-436

[35] Park Y, Hwang HB, Kim HS. Observation of influence of cataract surgery on the ocular surface. PLoS One. 2016;**11**(10):e0152460-e0152460

[36] Kim JS et al. Assessment of the tear film lipid layer thickness after cataract

surgery. Seminars in Ophthalmology. 2018;**33**(2):231-236

[37] Elksnis Ē et al. Tear osmolarity after cataract surgery. Journal of Current Ophthalmology. 2018;**31**(1):31-35

[38] González-Mesa A et al. Role of tear Osmolarity in dry eye symptoms after cataract surgery. American Journal of Ophthalmology. 2016;**170**:128-132

[39] Norn M. Quantitative tear ferning. Clinical Investigations. Acta Ophthalmologica (Copenh). 1994;**72**(3):369-372

[40] Qiu JJ et al. A study of dry eye after cataract surgery in MGD patients. International Ophthalmology. 2020;**40**(5):1277-1284

[41] Oh T et al. Changes in the tear film and ocular surface after cataract surgery. Japanese Journal of Ophthalmology. 2012;**56**(2):113-118

[42] Li XM et al. Investigation of dry eye disease and analysis of the pathogenic factors in patients after cataract surgery. Cornea. 2007;**26**(9 Suppl 1):S16-S20

[43] Zamora MG, Caballero EF, Maldonado MJ. Short-term changes in ocular surface signs and symptoms after phacoemulsification. European Journal of Ophthalmology. Nov 2020;**30**(6):1301-1307

[44] Khanal S et al. Changes in corneal sensitivity and tear physiology after phacoemulsification. Ophthalmic and Physiological Optics. 2008;**28**(2):127-134

[45] Ju R-H et al. Changes in ocular surface status and dry eye symptoms following femtosecond laser-assisted cataract surgery. International Journal of Ophthalmology. 2019;**12**(7):1122-1126

[46] Shao D et al. Effects of femtosecond laser-assisted cataract surgery on dry eye. Experimental and Therapeutic Medicine. 2018;**16**(6):5073-5078

[47] Hua H et al. Evaluation of dry eye after femtosecond laser-assisted cataract surgery. Journal of Cataract and Refractive Surgery. 2015;**41**(12):2614-2623

[48] Schargus M, Ivanova S, Stute G, Dick HB, Joachim SC. Comparable effects on tear film parameters after femtosecond laser-assisted and conventional cataract surgery. International Ophthalmology. Nov 2020;**40**(11):3097-3104

[49] Zhang Y et al. Alteration of tear film after sutureless large incision manual cataract extraction. International Journal of Ophthalmology. 2010;**10**(1):18-20

[50] Dasgupta S, Gupta R. The course of dry eye following phacoemulsification and manual-SICS: A prospective study based on Indian scenario. International Eye Science. 2016;**16**(10):1789-1794

[51] Garg P et al. Dry eye disease after cataract surgery: Study of its determinants and risk factors. Turkish Journal of Ophthalmology. 2020;**50**(3):133-142

[52] Kim EY, Kim MH, Yang HS. Change of the tear film instability and subjective symptoms after small-incision cataract surgery. Journal of the Korean Ophthalmological Society. 2012;**53**(9):1269-1275

[53] Venugopal KC, Krishnaraj PA, Chandan N. Evaluation of dryness of eyes after manual small incision cataract surgery with corneoscleral tunnel incision. Journal of Clinical and Diagnostic Research. 2012;**6**(6):1029-1033

[54] Jiang D et al. Transient tear film dysfunction after cataract surgery in diabetic patients. PLoS One. 2016;**11**(1):e0146752-e0146752

[55] Ram J et al. Cataract surgery in patients with dry eyes. Journal of Cataract and Refractive Surgery. 1998;**24**(8):1119-1124

[56] Sajnani R et al. Epidemiology of persistent postsurgical pain manifesting as dry eye-like symptoms after cataract surgery. Cornea. 2018;**37**(12):1535-1541

[57] Iglesias E et al. Epidemiology of persistent dry eye-like symptoms after cataract surgery. Cornea. 2018;**37**(7):893-898

[58] Min JS et al. Relationship between dry eye symptoms after cataract surgery and psychiatric status. The Ocular Surface. 2022;**23**:201-203

[59] Kumar CM, Eid H, Dodds C. Sub-Tenon's anaesthesia: Complications and their prevention. Eye (London, England). 2011;**25**(6):694-703

[60] Mimura T et al. Changes of conjunctivochalasis after cataract surgery via a superior transconjunctival sclerocorneal incision. International Ophthalmology. 2017;**37**(3):691-700

[61] Starr CE et al. An algorithm for the preoperative diagnosis and treatment of ocular surface disorders. Journal of Cataract and Refractive Surgery. 2019;**45**(5):669-684

[62] Villani E et al. The ocular surface frailty index as a predictor of ocular surface symptom onset after cataract surgery. Ophthalmology. 2020;**127**(7):866-873

[63] Gupta PK et al. Prevalence of ocular surface dysfunction in patients presenting for cataract surgery evaluation. Journal of Cataract and Refractive Surgery. 2018;**44**(9):1090-1096

[64] Epitropoulos AT et al. Effect of tear osmolarity on repeatability of keratometry for cataract surgery planning. Journal of Cataract and Refractive Surgery. 2015;**41**(8):1672-1677

[65] Kim P, Plugfelder S, Slomovic AR. Top 5 pearls to consider when implanting advanced-technology IOLs in patients with ocular surface disease. International Ophthalmology Clinics. 2012;**52**(2):51-58

[66] Salouti R et al. Comparison of the ultrasonographic method with 2 partial coherence interferometry methods for intraocular lens power calculation. Optometry - Journal of the American Optometric Association. 2011;**82**(3):140-147

[67] Röggla V et al. Influence of artificial tears on Keratometric measurements in cataract patients. American Journal of Ophthalmology. 2021;**221**:1-8

[68] Biela K et al. Dry eye disease as a cause of refractive errors after cataract surgery - a systematic review. Clinical Ophthalmology. 2023;**17**:1629-1638

[69] Teshigawara T, Meguro A, Mizuki N. The effect of Rebamipide on refractive accuracy of cataract surgery in patients with dry eye. Ophthalmology and Therapy. 2022;**11**(2):603-611

[70] Buznego C, Trattler WB. Presbyopia-correcting intraocular lenses. Current Opinion in Ophthalmology. 2009;**20**(1):13-18

[71] Lee JH, Kim JH, Kim SW. Repeatability of central corneal thickness measurement using rotating Scheimpflug

camera in dry and Normal eyes. Eye & Contact Lens. 2018;**44**(Suppl 2):S29-s32

[72] Çakır B et al. Effects of artificial tear treatment on corneal epithelial thickness and corneal topography findings in dry eye patients. Journal Français d'Ophtalmologie. 2018;**41**(5):407-411

[73] Chantra S, Jamtubtim S. Effects of dry eyes on corneal keratometry measured by VERIONTM image guided system. Journal of the Medical Association of Thailand. 2018;**101**(2 Supplement 2):S115-S121

[74] Song P et al. Preoperative management of MGD alleviates the aggravation of MGD and dry eye induced by cataract surgery: A prospective. Randomized Clinical Trial. Biomed Res Int. 2019;**2019**:2737968

[75] Favuzza E et al. Protecting the ocular surface in cataract surgery: The efficacy of the perioperative use of a hydroxypropyl guar and hyaluronic acid ophthalmic solution. Clinical Ophthalmology. 2020;**14**:1769-1775

[76] Fogagnolo P et al. New therapeutic strategy and innovative lubricating ophthalmic solution in minimizing dry eye disease associated with cataract surgery: A randomized, prospective study. Advances in Therapy. 2020;**37**(4):1664-1674

[77] Donnenfeld ED et al. Cyclosporine 0.05% to improve visual outcomes after multifocal intraocular lens implantation. Journal of Cataract and Refractive Surgery. 2010;**36**(7):1095-1100

[78] Ganesh S, Brar S, Bagare SN. Topical cyclosporine (0.05%) for management of dry eyes in patients undergoing cataract surgery-a comparative study. Open Ophthalmology Journal. 2019;**13**(1):34-42

[79] Shokoohi-Rad S et al. Effects of preoperative doses of betamethasone acetate 0.1% on dry eye control after cataract surgery. Indian Journal of Ophthalmology. 2020;**68**(3):450-454

[80] Lee H et al. Effect of diquafosol three per cent ophthalmic solution on tear film and corneal aberrations after cataract surgery. Clinical & Experimental Optometry. 2017;**100**(6):590-594

[81] Ge J et al. Evaluation of the efficacy of optimal pulsed technology treatment in patients with cataract and Meibomian gland dysfunction in the perioperative period. BMC Ophthalmology. 2020;**20**(1):111

[82] Ram J et al. Outcomes of phacoemulsification in patients with dry eye. Journal of Cataract and Refractive Surgery. 2002;**28**(8):1386-1389

[83] Yoshida A et al. Apoptosis in perforated cornea of a patient with graft-versus-host disease. Canadian Journal of Ophthalmology. 2006;**41**(4):472-475

[84] Nassiri N et al. Ocular graft versus host disease following allogeneic stem cell transplantation: A review of current knowledge and recommendations. Journal of Ophthalmic & Vision Research. 2013;**8**(4):351-358

[85] Balaram M, Dana MR. Phacoemulsification in patients after allogeneic bone marrow transplantation. Ophthalmology. 2001;**108**(9):1682-1687

[86] de Melo Franco R et al. Outcomes of cataract surgery in graft-versus-host disease. Cornea. 2015;**34**(5):506-511

[87] Penn EA, Soong KH. Cataract surgery in allogeneic bone marrow transplant recipients with graft-versus-host disease. Journal of Cataract & Refractive Surgery. 2002;**28**(3):417-420

[88] Shah A, Santhiago MR, Espana EM. Cataract surgery in patients with chronic severe graft-versus-host disease. Journal of Cataract and Refractive Surgery. 2016;**42**(6):833-839

[89] Sangwan VS, Burman S. Cataract surgery in Stevens-Johnson syndrome. Journal of Cataract & Refractive Surgery. 2005;**31**(4):860-862

[90] Narang P et al. Cataract surgery in chronic Stevens-Johnson syndrome: Aspects and outcomes. The British Journal of Ophthalmology. 2016;**100**(11):1542-1546

[91] Waheeb S. Topical anesthesia in phacoemulsification. Oman Journal of Ophthalmology. 2010;**3**(3):136-139

[92] Chandra S et al. The effectiveness of 2% lidocaine gel compared to 0.5% tetracaine eye drop as topical anesthetic agent for phacoemulsification surgery. Anesthesiology and Pain Medicine. 2018;**8**(2):e68383

[93] Marqués-Fernández V et al. An objective evaluation of the upper eyelid position after phacoemulsification cataract surgery. Seminars in Ophthalmology. 2019;**34**(6):442-445

[94] Moon H et al. Short-term influence of aspirating speculum use on dry eye after cataract surgery: A prospective study. Cornea. 2014;**33**(4):373-375

[95] Lafosse E et al. Presbyopia and the aging eye: Existing refractive approaches and their potential impact on dry eye signs and symptoms. Contact Lens & Anterior Eye. 2020;**43**(2):103-114

[96] He Y et al. The improvement of dry eye after cataract surgery by intraoperative using ophthalmic viscosurgical devices on the surface of cornea: The results of a consort-compliant randomized controlled trial. Medicine (Baltimore). 2017;**96**(50):e8940

[97] El-Harazi SM, Feldman RM. Control of intra-ocular inflammation associated with cataract surgery. Current Opinion in Ophthalmology. 2001;**12**(1):4-8

[98] Yusufu M et al. Hydroxypropyl methylcellulose 2% for dry eye prevention during phacoemulsification in senile and diabetic patients. International Ophthalmology. 2018;**38**(3):1261-1273

[99] Mencucci R et al. Triphasic polymeric corneal coating gel versus a balanced salt solution irrigation during cataract surgery: A postoperative anterior segment optical coherence tomography analysis and confocal microscopy evaluation. Journal of Cataract and Refractive Surgery. 2019;**45**(8):1148-1155

[100] Yoon DY et al. Evaluation of the protective effect of an ophthalmic Viscosurgical device on the ocular surface in dry eye patients during cataract surgery. Korean Journal of Ophthalmology. 2019;**33**(5):467-474

[101] Belmonte C, Acosta MC, Gallar J. Neural basis of sensation in intact and injured corneas. Experimental Eye Research. 2004;**78**(3):513-525

[102] The definition and classification of dry eye disease. Report of the definition and classification Subcommittee of the International dry eye WorkShop (2007). The Ocular Surface. 2007;**5**(2):75-92

[103] Dastjerdi MH, Dana R. Corneal nerve alterations in dry eye-associated ocular surface disease. International Ophthalmology Clinics. 2009;**49**(1):11-20

[104] Cho YK, Kim MS. Dry eye after cataract surgery and associated

intraoperative risk factors. Korean Journal of Ophthalmology. 2009;**23**(2):65-73

[105] Kohlhaas M. Corneal sensation after cataract and refractive surgery. Journal of Cataract and Refractive Surgery. 1998;**24**(10):1399-1409

[106] Sahu PK et al. Dry eye following phacoemulsification surgery and its relation to associated intraoperative risk factors. Middle East African Journal of Ophthalmology. 2015;**22**(4):472-477

[107] Donnenfeld ED, Solomon KD, Matossian C. Safety of IBI-10090 for inflammation associated with cataract surgery: Phase 3 multicenter study. Journal of Cataract and Refractive Surgery. 2018;**44**(10):1236-1246

[108] Donnenfeld E, Holland E. Dexamethasone Intracameral drug-delivery suspension for inflammation associated with cataract surgery: A randomized, placebo-controlled, Phase III Trial. Ophthalmology. 2018;**125**(6):799-806

[109] Chen X et al. Efficacy of an ocular bandage contact lens for the treatment of dry eye after phacoemulsification. BMC Ophthalmology. 2019;**19**(1):13-13

[110] Tyson SL et al. Multicenter randomized phase 3 study of a sustained-release intracanalicular dexamethasone insert for treatment of ocular inflammation and pain after cataract surgery. Journal of Cataract and Refractive Surgery. 2019;**45**(2):204-212

[111] Walters T et al. Sustained-release dexamethasone for the treatment of ocular inflammation and pain after cataract surgery. Journal of Cataract and Refractive Surgery. 2015;**41**(10):2049-2059

[112] Jee D et al. Comparison of treatment with preservative-free versus preserved sodium hyaluronate 0.1% and fluorometholone 0.1% eyedrops after cataract surgery in patients with preexisting dry-eye syndrome. Journal of Cataract and Refractive Surgery. 2015;**41**(4):756-763

[113] Chung YW, Oh TH, Chung SK. The effect of topical cyclosporine 0.05% on dry eye after cataract surgery. Korean Journal of Ophthalmology. 2013;**27**(3):167-171

[114] Kudyar P et al. Comparative evaluation of efficacy and safety of cyclosporine 0.1% add-on therapy with artificial tears (carboxymethylcellulose 0.5%) with artificial tears alone in post cataract surgery patients. National Journal of Physiology, Pharmacy and Pharmacology. 2018;**8**(12):1685-1691

[115] Baek J, Doh SH, Chung SK. The effect of topical Diquafosol Tetrasodium 3% on dry eye after cataract surgery. Current Eye Research. 2016;**41**(10):1281-1285

[116] Cui L et al. Effect of diquafosol tetrasodium 3% on the conjunctival surface and clinical findings after cataract surgery in patients with dry eye. International Ophthalmology. 2018;**38**(5):2021-2030

[117] Miyake K, Yokoi N. Influence on ocular surface after cataract surgery and effect of topical diquafosol on postoperative dry eye: A multicenter prospective randomized study. Clinical Ophthalmology. 2017;**11**:529-540

[118] Park DH et al. Clinical effects and safety of 3% Diquafosol ophthalmic solution for patients with dry eye after cataract surgery: A randomized controlled trial. American Journal of Ophthalmology. 2016;**163**:122-131.e2

[119] Jun I et al. Effects of preservative-free 3% Diquafosol in patients with pre-existing dry eye disease after cataract surgery: A randomized clinical trial. Scientific Reports. 2019;**9**(1):12659

[120] Lee JH et al. Effectiveness and optical quality of topical 3.0% Diquafosol versus 0.05% cyclosporine a in dry eye patients following cataract surgery. Journal of Ophthalmology. 2016;**2016**:8150757

[121] Inoue Y, Ochi S. Effects of 3% diquafosol sodium ophthalmic solution on higher-order aberrations in patients diagnosed with dry eye after cataract surgery. Clinical Ophthalmology. 2017;**11**:87-93

[122] Kato K et al. Conjunctival goblet cell density following cataract surgery with diclofenac versus diclofenac and Rebamipide: A randomized trial. American Journal of Ophthalmology. 2017;**181**:26-36

[123] Yao K et al. Efficacy of 1% carboxymethylcellulose sodium for treating dry eye after phacoemulsification: Results from a multicenter, open-label, randomized, controlled study. BMC Ophthalmology. 2015;**15**:28

[124] Mencucci R et al. Effect of a hyaluronic acid and carboxymethylcellulose ophthalmic solution on ocular comfort and tear-film instability after cataract surgery. Journal of Cataract and Refractive Surgery. 2015;**41**(8):1699-1704

[125] Caretti L et al. Efficacy of carbomer sodium hyaluronate trehalose vs hyaluronic acid to improve tear film instability and ocular surface discomfort after cataract surgery. Clinical Ophthalmology. 2019;**13**:1157-1163

[126] Mohammadpour M, Maleki S, Khorrami-Nejad M. The effect of tea tree oil on dry eye treatment after phacoemulsification cataract surgery: A randomized clinical trial. European Journal of Ophthalmology. Nov 2020;**30**(6):1314-1319

[127] Mohammadpour M et al. Effects of adjuvant omega-3 fatty acid supplementation on dry eye syndrome following cataract surgery: A randomized clinical trial. Journal of Current Ophthalmology. 2017;**29**(1):33-38

[128] Park J, Yoo YS, Shin E, Han G, Shin K, Lim DH, et al. Effects of the re-esterified triglyceride (rTG) form of omega-3 supplements on dry eye following cataract surgery. The British Journal of Ophthalmology. Nov 2021;**105**(11):1504-1509

[129] Son HS et al. Semi-fluorinated alkane eye drops reduce signs and symptoms of evaporative dry eye disease after cataract surgery. Journal of Refractive Surgery. 2020;**36**(7):474-480

[130] Devendra J, Singh S. Effect of Oral Lactoferrin on cataract surgery induced dry eye: A randomised controlled trial. Journal of Clinical and Diagnostic Research. 2015;**9**(10):Nc06-9

Chapter 4

Evolution of Biometric Formulas and Intraocular Lens Selection in Challenging Cases

Ezgi Karataş and Canan Aslı Utine

Abstract

Various novel intraocular lens (IOL) power calculation formulas have been described to increase refractive precision following cataract surgery. These include the Barrett Universal II, Emmetropia Verifying Optical (EVO), Kane, Naeser 2, Olsen, Panacea, Pearl DGS, Radial Basis Function (RBF), T2, and VRF formulas. With a few notable exceptions, historical and regression formulas—first- and second-generation IOL formulas like Sanders, Retzlaff, Kraff (SRK), Binkhorst, Hoffer, and SRKII—are generally regarded as outdated. The effective lens position (ELP) is accounted for in third- and fourth-generation formulas which include more biometric data. A possible alternative that has shown to be remarkably accurate when used with the Olsen method is ray tracing. Artificial intelligence-derived IOL formulas are becoming increasingly common and may yield better lens power prediction accuracy. Despite improvements in surgical technique, biometry measurements, and IOL calculations, some clinical circumstances continue to challenge cataract surgeons to determine the appropriate IOL power. These unique situations include pediatric eyes, post-refractive eyes, and corneal ectasias. The obstacles to reliability include unrepeatable measurements and inaccurate biometry examinations. Researchers have tried to identify the most accurate IOL estimations for these challenging clinical scenarios to overcome these obstacles.

Keywords: artificial intelligence, biometry, ectasia, post-refractive surgery, ray tracing, vergence formulas

1. Introduction

The development of biometric criteria for choosing appropriate intraocular lens (IOL) power has been continuous. The power of the IOL that will be placed after cataract surgery is determined using biometric formulas. The objective is to provide the patient with the best visual result possible. Aiming for residual hyperopia, employing the Haigis formula for biometric calculation, or applying a customized surgeon's A-constant are just a few of the ways previously recommended by authors to address the errors in IOL power assessment [1]. Artificial intelligence has been used in recent biometric formula innovations. Various generations of formulas have been developed to choose the IOL dioptric power as a function of its anticipated postoperative

IntechOpen

position. However, only a minority of formulas—usually one-dimensional—include information about crystalline lenses [2].

2. Evolution of formulas

2.1 Empiric formulas

The Sanders-Retzlaff-Kraff (SRK I, SRK II) formulas, the first to represent a statistical regression technique, were reported to produce better results than early theoretical formulas in the early years of IOL power computation. Any empirical approach has the benefit of being based on actual measurements, which reduces the need for assumptions. For instance, how to calculate corneal power, account for principal planes, correct axial length for retinal thickness, and make any clinical measurements work in the physical sense. A regression formula functions by generating a mean value and accounting for departures from the mean using regression coefficients. The mathematical mean errors of a regression equation should accumulate to zero in a representative patient sample if it is correctly derived [3].

The first formula of SRK I was a straightforward linear regression equation: $P = A - 2.5AL - 0.9\,K$ where AL = the axial length of the eye as measured by ultrasound, P0 = the power of the implant for emmetropia, K = the dioptric keratometry reading (using index 1.3375), A = the A-constant according to the kind of IOL, and the mean values of the K-readings and axial length readings.

Any empirical approach has the drawback that, in theory, its formula only applies to the dataset from which it was developed. For instance, the A-constant (and perhaps the regression coefficients) will change if the axial length is assessed using a different method in a different clinical situation. This would be the case when switching from ultrasound to partial coherence interferometry (PCI) (Carl Zeiss Meditec, Jena, Germany), which tends to provide longer readings than ultrasound. The formula, however, may also be susceptible to variations in surgical technique, such as whether the IOL is positioned inside or outside the capsular bag, which can change the IOL's average location and refractive effect.

2.2 Theoretical formulas

They have a Gaussian optics foundation. This theoretical formula contains six variables, which are

1. Net corneal power (K)

2. Axial length (AL)

3. IOL power (IOLP)

4. Effective lens position (ELP)

5. Refraction desired (D Post Rx)

6. Vertex distance (V) [4]

2.2.1 First generation

The anterior chamber depth (ACD) was presumed to be constant for all eyes in the first generation of theoretical formulations for intraocular lenses, which included the Binkhorst I, Fyodorov, and Colenbrander formulas. These calculations were inaccurate for all eyes because they were built on the simplistic assumption that the ACD had a set value [5].

2.2.2 Second generation

They refer to specific theoretical or regression formulas. Intraocular lens formulas from the first generation were correct in eyes with standard lengths, but they struggled in eyes that were unusually long or short. As a result, the formula needed to be changed for the axial length to be factored correctly. The original SRK formula, $P = A - 2.5\,L - 0.9\,K + C$, was modified to create the SRK II or second-generation regression formula. Regression analysis of the postoperative refractive error in numerous eyes was used to calculate the C-value [4]. Regression investigation of the postoperative refractive error in many eyes yielded the C-value in the SRK II calculation. The C-value is 3 for an axial length of 10–20 mm. The C-value is 2.0 if the axial length is 20–21 mm. The C-value is 1 for 21–22 mm. It is 0 for 22–24.5 mm. The C-value is −0.5 if the axial length is more than 24.5. In conclusion, the SRK II and other second-generation intraocular lens formulas employed the C-value to modify the formula so that the axial length could be precisely factored. Other formulas used the observed axial length, such as the modified Binkhorst Formula and Hoffer's ACD Adjustment [6].

2.2.3 Third generation

By accounting for unique differences in the position and shape of the crystalline lens, third-generation intraocular lens formulas have been created to increase the precision of IOL power estimation. The Holladay 1, Hoffer Q, and Sanders-Retzlaff-Kraff/Theoretical (i.e., SRK/T) formulas are examples of these formulas. Note that the SRK/T formula is the most recent version of SRK formulas. It is not a regression formula but a modified Binkhorst model with changed anterior chamber depth (ACD)-prediction algorithms. The third-generation intraocular lens formulas have been found to estimate IOL power more accurately than the first- and second-generation formulas [7–9].

The axial length, corneal power, and anterior chamber depth are used in the Holladay 1 formula to determine the IOL power. To increase the accuracy of IOL power estimation, the Holladay 2 formula adds the surgeon factor and lens thickness to the Holladay 1 method. The Hoffer Q formula, which calculates IOL power using the axial length, corneal power, and ACD, has been determined to be the most accurate method for doing so in eyes with axial lengths less than 22 mm. The best precise formula for calculating IOL power in eyes with axial lengths more than 22 mm is the SRK/T formula, which uses the axial length, corneal power, and ACD.

2.2.4 Fourth generation

These formulas have been utilized in numerous research and were created to increase the precision of IOL power calculations. The Holladay 2 technique is a formula that takes seven factors into account, including age, axial length (AL), keratometry, anterior chamber depth (ACD), white-to-white measurement, and lens thickness (LT). In short eyes (22 mm), the Holladay 2 formula is reliable for forecasting IOL power. Holladay 2 was more accurate than Holladay 1 and equal to Hoffer Q in short eyes <22.0 mm [10].

The Haigis formula was developed in 2000 to calculate the power of intraocular lenses (IOLs). It uses three independent constants called a0, a1, and a2 to predict IOL power. These constants, unique to the formula, are determined from regression analysis of clinical data. All three constants can be adjusted using linear regression to improve the function's ability to predict outcomes accurately. In long eyes (>26 mm), the Haigis formula is reliable for forecasting IOL power [11].

2.2.5 New novel formulas

The Barrett Universal II formula is an IOL power calculation formula introduced in 2014 to modify the original Barrett Universal formula. It uses biometric parameters, including axial length, keratometry, anterior chamber depth, and lens thickness, to predict IOL power. The accuracy of the Barrett Universal II formula has been studied in various populations, including post-corneal refractive surgery eyes, highly myopic patients, and pediatric cataract patients with multifocal IOL implantation. The formula has produced better refractive outcomes than other formulas in some studies [12]. This formula has also been used in studies evaluating the efficacy of different IOLs, such as trifocal presbyopia-correcting IOLs and non-diffractive extended depth of focus or neutral aspheric monofocal IOLs [13].

The Barrett Universal II formula provides better predictability of IOL power calculation. It is less susceptible to the effect of the axial length and the corneal shape than the SRK/T formula in eyes requiring combined cataract surgery and trabeculectomy [14].

Emmetropia Verifying Optical (EVO) is a technology used in intraocular lens (IOL) power calculation to verify the accuracy of the selected IOL power. EVO uses a wavefront aberrometer to measure the patient's postoperative refraction and compare it to the predicted refraction based on the desired IOL power. The desired IOL power is considered accurate if the measured refraction is within a specific range of the expected refraction. If the measured refraction exceeds this range, the EVO technology can suggest a different IOL power to achieve the desired refractive outcome. EVO can be used in both cataract surgery and refractive lens exchange procedures. Using EVO can improve the accuracy of IOL power calculation and reduce the need for postoperative refractive adjustments. However, EVO is not widely available and may only be necessary in some cases, particularly in patients with normal ocular anatomy and biometry. In conclusion, Emmetropia Verifying Optical (EVO) is a technology used in IOL power calculation to verify the accuracy of the selected IOL power. Its use can improve the accuracy of IOL power calculation and reduce the need for postoperative refractive adjustments, but it may not be necessary in all cases [15].

Based on theoretical optics, the new Kane formula (found at www.iolformula.com) also integrates regression and artificial intelligence to improve its predictions further. The Kane formula is a widely used IOL power calculation formula that accurately predicts IOL power in various populations. To anticipate the refractive result, it considers the patient's gender, axial length, keratometry, anterior chamber depth, lens thickness, and central corneal thickness [16]. In several studies, the Kane formula had a higher percentage of eyes within ±0.25 D of the predicted refraction than other formulas, including the Hoffer Q, SRK/T, and Holladay 1 formulas. The Kane formula also had the highest percentage of eyes within ±0.25D and ±1.00D in a comparison study of 13 formulas [17]. The Kane keratoconus formula was the most accurate in a study of patients with keratoconus [18]. The Kane formula was also accurate in vitrectomized eyes and eyes with high axial myopia [19]. In a study of sharp eyes, the Kane formula had a statistically significantly lower mean absolute error compared to all other formulas except the EVO 2.0 [20].

The Naeser 2 formula was developed by Naeser in 1997. It is based on vergence calculation and lens design and uses two keratometry readings, axial length, and anterior chamber depth, to predict IOL power. The Naeser 2 formula has been studied in various populations and accurately predicts IOL power. In a study of patients older than 80 years with cataracts and corneal astigmatism, the Naeser-Savini formula achieved the lowest mean absolute error and had the highest percentages of eyes within an absolute error of 0.50 D and 1.00 D compared to other formulas [21]. However, the Naeser formula has not been widely studied compared to other formulas, and its accuracy has yet been proven from empirical data. Further research is needed to determine its efficacy as compared to other formulas.

The Olsen formula uses ray tracing technology to predict IOL power. It considers the individual optical properties of the cornea, lens, and eye axial length to calculate the optimal IOL power. The Olsen formula has been studied in various populations and accurately predicts IOL power [22]. In a study comparing the Olsen formula to other formulas, the Olsen formula had the lowest mean absolute error and the highest percentage of eyes within ±0.50 D of the predicted refraction [23]. The Olsen formula has also been found to be accurate in eyes with high myopia and eyes with previous corneal refractive surgery [24, 25].

The Panacea formula, created by David Flikier, is a vergence formula that includes the precise measurement of anterior and posterior corneal curvature data to establish and use total corneal astigmatism [26]. This formula can be accessed from the Panacea IOL and Toric calculator software (www.panaceaiolandtoriccalculator.com). The Panacea formula does not mathematically calculate the posterior corneal surface from the anterior surface. It takes into account the actual values of the anterior and posterior surfaces to provide the total corneal astigmatism, which generates more accurate calculations [27]. It is a thin-lens vergence formula with the unique possibility of including the anterior-to-posterior corneal curvature ratio and the asphericity (Q value at 6.0 mm) of the anterior corneal surface [28].

A more contemporary formula, the Pearl-DGS, was created by G. Debellemanière, D. Gatinel, et al. Optical and machine learning models were used to create this unpublished formula. AI-enhanced prediction and output linearization are used, and the A-constant from the SRK/T formula is necessary. This formula may be found at http://www.iolsolver.com [28].

2.2.5.1 Radial basis function 2.0

This AI-based algorithm calculates the IOL power using the radial basis function. It is available online at http://www.rbfcalculator.com [28]. Radial basis function methods are not limited to IOL power calculation. It has been used in various fields, including function interpolation, hyperspectral data classification, and artificial neural networks.

The formula has been studied in various populations and accurately predicts IOL power. In a study comparing the Hill-Radial Basis Function 2.0 formula to the Barrett Universal II formula and the SRK/T formula, the Hill-Radial Basis Function 2.0 formula had similar accuracy to the other formulas [29]. In another study comparing to other artificial intelligence-based formulas, including the Kane and PEARL-DGS formulas, the Hill-Radial Basis Function 2.0 formula had similar or better accuracy than the other formulas [30]. The Hill-Radial Basis Function 2.0 formula has been accurate in eyes undergoing manual or femtosecond laser-assisted cataract surgery.

The T2 formula was created to enhance the SRK/T formula's original design. Excel was programmed with the actual data in mind. For postoperative prediction of the anterior eye portion, it uses the same optical A-constant of the SRK/T and an upgraded regression algorithm [28]. However, further research is needed to determine its efficacy compared to other formulas in different populations.

2.2.5.2 VRF

This vergence-based thin-lens formula uses the optical CACD constant and four variables to determine the IOL power: AL, K, ACD, and the horizontal CD. The author programmed it into Excel [28]. In a study comparing the VRF-G formula to other formulas, including the Kane, Hoffer QST, and Barrett Universal II formulas, the VRF-G formula was more accurate than older formulas. The VRF-G formula had a standard deviation of ±0.387 D, which was lower than the standard deviations of the other formulas [31]. The VRF formula is unrelated to the other references, which discuss formulas and mathematical calculations in various fields, including medicine, engineering, and linguistics.

The Castrop intraocular lens (IOL) calculation formula is a recent development to evaluate the accuracy of IOL power calculation in patients with short axial eye length who are strong hyperopes. The Castrop formula is based on a pseudophakic model eye and has shown slightly superior performance to classical formulas such as the SRKT, Hoffer-Q, Holladay1, or Haigis formulas. The Castrop formula has not been published before but has been disclosed in a ready-to-use Excel sheet as an addendum to a research paper. The formula was evaluated in a single-center study in Germany that involved patients who underwent uneventful cataract surgery and were implanted with either spherical or aspheric IOLs. While the Castrop formula showed slightly superior performance compared to the classical formulas, future studies are needed to evaluate the reliability and accuracy of the formula. Further optimization of formula constants and consideration of variables such as keratometer or corneal refractive index in different IOL formulas can improve overall performance and accuracy in IOL power calculations [32–35].

At this juncture, it is necessary to briefly discuss the effect of anterior segment depth (ASD) on residual refraction after cataract surgery. The ASD, i.e., the sum of the anterior chamber depth and lens thickness, can affect the accuracy of IOL calculation formulas. Kesim et al. found that different ASD measurements affect the accuracy of seven different IOL calculation formulas, with larger ASD leading to higher mean absolute error values [36]. Positive correlations were found between ASD and the predictive errors of the SRK/T, Holladay I, Hoffer Q, Barrett II, Hill-RBF, and Haigis formulas. In cases with mean K greater than 42,0 D, ASD was similarly correlated with PE, except for the Olsen OLCR formula. In eyes with an AL between 22.5 and 24.5 mm, the predictions of lens formulas were substantially hyperopic in cases with greater ASD, according to their findings. Overall, the accuracy of IOL power calculations depends on many factors, including ASD, axial length, keratometry, and individual patient characteristics, which should be considered when selecting the appropriate IOL formula.

3. The approach in challenging cataract cases

3.1 Pediatric eyes

Pediatric cataract is a leading cause of childhood blindness, and their management can be challenging due to the growing size of the affected eyes and the risk of amblyopia. The etiology of pediatric cataracts varies and can be classified according to their time of onset, morphology, and underlying cause. The most common etiology of pediatric cataracts is idiopathic, meaning the reason is unknown. However, genetic factors play a role in the development of congenital cataracts, and genetic counseling and molecular testing should be undertaken in cases of hereditary cataracts. Other etiologies of pediatric cataracts include trauma, infections, metabolic disorders, and syndromes. Early diagnosis and treatment of pediatric cataracts are essential for good visual outcomes, and identifying the etiology of cataracts is necessary for counseling and preventive public programs.

A thorough ocular examination is essential in evaluating pediatric cataracts, including the onset, duration, and morphology of the cataract. Ocular malformations such as microphthalmos/microcornea are frequently associated with pediatric cataracts. The management of pediatric cataracts is a team effort involving ophthalmologists, pediatricians, anesthetists, and parents. It should be customized depending on the age of onset, laterality, the morphology of the cataract, and other associated ocular and systemic comorbidities. Newborns should be examined for ocular structural abnormalities, such as cataracts, corneal opacity, and ptosis, which are known to result in visual problems. Congenital cataracts and blunt ocular trauma are the most frequently observed congenital ocular disease and causes of ocular trauma among children. The frequency of strabismus and chronological, etiological, and morphological features should also be evaluated in patients with pediatric cataracts.

The decision to operate on pediatric cataracts depends on various factors, including the patient's age, the cataract's type and severity, and associated ocular and systemic comorbidities. Advances in surgical techniques and methods of optical rehabilitation have substantially improved the functional and anatomic outcomes of pediatric cataract surgeries in recent years. However, good visual outcomes require occlusion therapy and optical correction.

Pediatric cataract surgery is different from adult cataract surgery. It presents several intraoperative challenges, including low scleral rigidity, which makes it difficult to construct incisions and close wounds; the smaller size of the eyeball, shallow anterior chamber depth, and small pupil size, which reduces maneuverability; and an elastic capsule, which increases the risk of vitreous loss and expulsion of intraocular contents. The benefits of primary IOL implantation include quick postoperative refractive correction, minor to no optical aberration, an entire visual field, a reduced risk of amblyopia onset and progression, and little reliance on patient compliance. IOL implantation in children under the age of two is still debatable. The primary reasons for the limited use of IOL implantation in children under two years of age include the lack of long-term data to predict the success rate, linked additional ocular problems with cataracts, systematic development of deprivation amblyopia, and increased postoperative morbidity.

3.2 Surgical technique

3.2.1 Anterior capsule management

Pediatric cataract therapy relies heavily on anterior curvilinear capsulorhexis (CCC) since it chooses the surgical approach and location of the IOL fixation. Since the anterior capsule in children is relatively elastic, a controlled manual CCC may be challenging. The rhexis margin is still the gold standard in strength, however. Therefore, a manual anterior continuous curvilinear capsulorhexis should be performed wherever possible. The size and shape of the anterior capsulotomy are crucial for the IOL to remain centered for a long time. Staining the anterior capsule with trypan blue 0.1% has been shown to allow recognition of capsule flaps and facilitate the creation of complete anterior CCC and posterior PCCC in pediatric cataract surgery. Indocyanine green (ICG) staining has been evaluated to enhance the visualization of the anterior lens capsule in dense pediatric, mature cataracts. Femtosecond laser-assisted capsulorhexis, vitrectorhexis, radiofrequency diathermy, and Fugo plasma blade-assisted rhexis are options for manual CCC.

3.2.2 Management of the posterior capsule and anterior vitreous face

After juvenile cataract surgery, visual axis opacification (VAO) is the most prevalent and severe issue. Significant VAO in children hinders recovery and development of the visual system. Amblyopia may also result from it. A primary posterior capsulotomy is therefore regarded as a "routine surgical step," particularly in young children up to the age of eight years (with or without anterior vitrectomy). The posterior capsulotomy procedure can be carried out using various techniques, including radiofrequency diathermy, the Fugo plasma blade, femtosecond laser-aided capsulorhexis, vitrectorhexis, and manual posterior CCC. In contrast, if a pars plana vitrectorhexis is performed, most surgeons prefer to execute it after IOL implantation. Most surgeons prefer to perform manual posterior CCC before IOL implantation. Nevertheless, it entirely depends on the surgeon's judgment and preferences [37].

Although it can be postponed, posterior CCC cannot prevent visual axis obscuration alone. The proliferating lens epithelial cells might use the anterior vitreous face (AVF) as a scaffold. Additionally, due to the severity of the inflammatory reaction in young children, fibrous membranes may develop on the intact AVF, leading to VAO. Therefore, a posterior capsulotomy and anterior vitrectomy are recommended for newborns and young children. In infants under the age of four, an anterior-posterior capsulotomy with anterior vitrectomy is preferred, whereas, in patients aged four to eight, only posterior capsulotomy is performed without anterior vitrectomy. However, some surgeons favor performing anterior vitrectomy on patients as young as six to seven.

3.2.3 Primary IOL implantation

Several studies have shown that primary IOL implantation can be a safe and effective option for treating pediatric cataracts, with outcomes comparable to contact lens correction or secondary IOL implantation. One study compared the visual outcomes of primary IOL implantation versus contact lens correction in children with unilateral congenital cataracts. The study found that both groups had similar visual outcomes in the first year of age [38]. Another study showed that at a 4.5-year follow-up, infants who underwent primary IOL implantation or were treated with contact lenses had similar visual outcomes. However, pseudophakic children had a greater incidence of complications and second interventions than the contact lens group [39].

On the other hand, Infant Aphakia Treatment Study also revealed the complications of primary IOL implantation. It is a clinical trial designed to compare the visual outcomes of patients who received either contact or intraocular lenses after cataract surgery during infancy. The study included 114 infants with unilateral congenital cataracts at 12 sites [40]. The study reported that after 4.8 years of surgery, the incidence of glaucoma and glaucoma plus glaucoma suspect in operated eyes for children up to age five years were 17 and 31%, respectively. However, neither the contact lens nor the IOL group had a significant difference in either outcome: glaucoma (hazard ratio HR, 0.8; 95% CI, 0.3–2.0; P = .62) and glaucoma + glaucoma suspect (HR, 1.3; 95% CI, 0.6–2.5; P = .58) [41]. Another study evaluated the outcomes of bilateral cataract surgery in infants aged one to seven months with Infant Aphakia Treatment Study (IATS) investigators and reported that 24% of children received primary IOL implantation, with a median visual acuity of 0.35 logarithm of the minimum angle of resolution in the better-seeing eye at the final study visit closest to five years of age [42]. The study also found that strabismus was detected in 81% of infants by age five [43]. Comparably, after 12 months of the follow-up, a secondary outcome analysis in a prospective, randomized clinical trial that included 114 infants with a unilateral congenital cataract, IOL, or contact lens replacement of the lens, observed a proportion of patients that developed strabismus [44]. However, the study found no significant difference in grating visual acuity between the IOL and contact lens groups [45]. The study observed patients up to five years old and found that both received similar visual outcomes [46].

In summary, the Infant Aphakia Treatment Study reported the frequency of different ocular conditions in infants after unilateral cataract surgery and the impact of different optical correction methods on visual outcomes. The study findings indicated that IOL implantation or contact lenses are suitable options for Infant Aphakia, with both alternatives having their risks and benefits.

Various techniques have been described for primary IOL implantation in pediatric cataracts, including posterior optic buttonholing, which involves implanting the IOL through the posterior capsulorhexis margin in cases of anterior capsulorhexis extension. This technique is feasible for children who experienced anterior capsulorhexis extension during pediatric cataract surgery, resulting in satisfactory surgical outcomes and few ocular complications [47].

In conclusion, primary IOL implantation may be a safe and effective option for treating pediatric cataracts, with outcomes comparable to contact lens correction or secondary IOL implantation in selected eyes. Various techniques and types of IOLs have been evaluated in different age groups and populations, and further studies are needed to determine the optimal approach for primary IOL implantation in pediatric cataracts.

3.2.4 Secondary IOL implantation

This technique involves the implantation of an IOL in the posterior chamber of the eye, either in the capsular bag or the ciliary sulcus. Several studies have evaluated the long-term visual outcomes and factors affecting visual results in children undergoing secondary IOL implantation following primary congenital cataract extraction. One study found that secondary IOL implantation resulted in good long-term visual outcomes in children with congenital cataracts [48]. Other studies have identified factors that may increase the risk of complications, such as secondary glaucoma, including high insertion of the iris and IOL implantation in the ciliary sulcus [49]. To reduce the risk of complications, researchers have modified the cataract extraction technique and secondary IOL implantation in pediatric aphakic eyes to achieve secondary in-the-bag IOL implantation [50]. However, the optimal size of the anterior capsulorhexis that should be used to obtain superior capsular outcomes for secondary IOL implantation in primary pediatric cataract surgery has yet to be reported [51].

Other studies have evaluated the safety and efficacy of different types of IOLs and techniques for secondary IOL implantation in pediatric cataracts. For example, posterior iris-fixated IOL implantation is an excellent alternative to other IOLs in pediatric traumatic cataracts without adequate capsular support [52]. Secondary PC-IOL implantation has also been effective in pediatric cataract eyes with microcornea and microphthalmos [53]. A recent multicenter, single-blinded, randomized controlled trial evaluated the safety and efficacy of in-the-bag versus sulcus fixation for secondary IOL implantation in pediatric cataract patients who have undergone primary cataract extraction. The study found that both techniques were safe and effective, with no significant differences in visual outcomes or complications between the two groups [54].

Various factors, such as the location of IOL implantation and the size of the anterior capsulorhexis, may affect the risk of complications. Further studies are needed to determine the optimal approach for secondary IOL implantation in pediatric cataracts.

3.2.5 IOL Power calculation in children

IOL power calculation is a crucial step in pediatric cataract surgery, as it determines the refractive outcome of the procedure. However, IOL power calculation in pediatric cataracts presents unique challenges due to the differences in ocular biometry and growth patterns compared to adults. Several studies have evaluated the accuracy of different IOL power calculation formulas and techniques in pediatric cataracts. New technologies for biometric measurements and keratometry in pediatric eyes have been developed to improve the accuracy of IOL power calculation.

Controversies in pediatric cataract management regarding the timing of surgery, IOL power calculation, and the choice of IOL still exist. Currently, the majority of surgeons prefer to use the SRK-T formula. One study compared the SRK-T, Holladay 1, Holladay 2, and Hoffer Q formulas and showed that SRK-T and Holladay 2 formulas have the lowest prediction error [55]. Young children develop myopia over time due to significant retina growth and corneal curvature changes. Therefore, many surgeons plan initial under-correction and provide refractive correction with contact lenses or spectacles [56, 57]. In cases of unilateral cataracts, fellow eye's refractive status, dense amblyopia, the likelihood of poor compliance, socioeconomic considerations for contact lens use, and individual surgeon practice patterns, however, surgeons tend to make the eye less hypermetropic. Further research is needed to improve the accuracy of IOL power calculation in pediatric cataracts.

3.3 High myopia

Cataract surgery in patients with severe pathologic myopia and high axial length is well documented. These patients often have a higher risk of complications such as retinal detachment, cystoid macular edema, and posterior capsular opacification. Patients face severe pathologic myopia and high axial length challenges during cataract surgery. Multiple studies have been conducted to evaluate the outcomes of cataract surgery in these patients.

According to the Beaver Dam Eye Study and the Blue Mountains Eye Study, myopia and nuclear cataract are associated. The Blue Mountains Eye Study also found that moderate and high myopia, particularly when it begins before age 20, is related to the formation of posterior subcapsular cataracts [58]. The Singapore Malay Eye Study also found that patients with severe myopia have a three to fivefold increased risk of nuclear cataracts and a 30% increased risk of posterior subcapsular cataracts [59].

Patients with severe pathologic myopia and high axial length are at risk of zonulopathy, which can be secondary to many pathologies, including mature cataracts, prior ocular trauma, or prior ocular surgery. Venkateswaran and Henderson reported that loose zonules could make cataract surgery more challenging in these patients [60]. Capsular or iris hooks, capsular tension rings, and capsular tension segments (CTS) are all viable options for capsular bag support in zonulopathy. Numerous surgical techniques for inserting these devices can be tailored to the surgeon's preference and the patient's eye morphology.

One of the significant risks associated with cataract surgery in high myopia patients is the presence of chorioretinal degenerations, which can lead to poor visual outcomes [61]. High myopia patients also have a higher risk of complications such as retinal detachment, cystoid macular edema, and posterior capsular opacification. These complications can lead to permanent vision loss and require additional treatment. Suprachoroidal hemorrhage (SCH) is another risk associated with cataract surgery in high myopia patients. Bozkurt and Miller reported a case of a patient with high myopia who developed an SCH at the time of cataract surgery following three femtosecond laser docking attempts [62]. Other risks associated with cataract surgery in high myopia patients include preexisting maculopathy or posterior staphyloma and early postoperative BCVA recovery risk factors [63]. Highly myopic cataract eyes are also at risk of low vision, and risk factors for low vision include younger age, longer axial length, and preexisting maculopathy.

Another risk associated with cataract surgery in high myopia patients is the variability of axial length, anterior chamber depth, and lens thickness [64]. This variability can make selecting the appropriate IOL power challenging, leading to postoperative refractive errors. Postoperative refractive errors can cause poor visual outcomes and require additional treatment.

Finally, high myopia patients undergoing cataract surgery may be at a higher risk of IOL dislocation, especially in younger patients [65]. Immediate sequential bilateral cataract surgery is another technique that may be associated with increased risks in high myopia patients [66].

In summary, high myopia patients undergoing cataract surgery are at a higher risk of complications and poor visual outcomes than emmetropic eyes. Therefore, careful monitoring and precautions should be taken to minimize the risks and improve postoperative outcomes in high myopia patients undergoing cataract surgery.

3.3.1 IOL calculations in high myopia

One of the main difficulties in IOL calculation in high myopia cataract patients is the accurate measurement of axial length (AL) and corneal curvature. High myopia patients often have longer AL, leading to errors in IOL power calculation if not adequately accounted for [67]. High myopia patients may have corneal astigmatism, further complicating IOL calculation [67]. Therefore, accurate AL and corneal curvature measurement is crucial for successful IOL calculation in high myopia cataract patients.

Another difficulty in IOL calculation in high myopia cataract patients is selecting the appropriate IOL design and power. Aspheric IOLs with low negative or zero primary spherical aberration are recommended for cataract patients with high myopia [68]. Negative power IOLs have also been used successfully in patients with extremely high myopia [69]. However, selecting the appropriate IOL design and power can be challenging due to the variability of axial length, anterior chamber depth, and lens thickness in high myopia eyes.

In addition, preexisting conditions such as posterior staphyloma, maculopathy, and photorefractive keratectomy (PRK) can further complicate IOL calculation in high myopia cataract patients. For example, PRK can alter the corneal curvature and affect the accuracy of IOL calculation [70]. Therefore, carefully considering preexisting conditions is necessary for successful IOL calculation in high myopia cataract patients. Furthermore, intraoperative aberrometry can help improve IOL calculation accuracy in high myopia cataract patients. Intraoperative aberrometry measures the eye's refractive error during surgery and can be used to adjust the IOL power accordingly [71]. However, intraoperative aberrometry may not be feasible in all cases and may add to the cost of the procedure.

In conclusion, IOL calculation in high myopia cataract patients can be challenging due to the unique anatomical and refractive characteristics of these eyes. Accurate measurement of axial length and corneal curvature, selection of the appropriate IOL design and power, consideration of preexisting conditions, and intraoperative aberrometry can contribute to successful IOL calculation in high myopia cataract patients. Therefore, careful planning and care of these factors are necessary for optimal outcomes in high myopia cataract surgery.

3.4 Hyperopia

The definition of a small eye is based on assessing ocular axial length (AL), anterior chamber depth (ACD), corneal diameter, and concomitant anatomical malformations. Simple microphthalmos is an eye with an AL shorter than the age-adjusted mean by two standard deviations, with a normal ACD, average scleral thickness, and without anatomical malformations. Nanophthalmos is a rare condition characterized by short AL with a shallow anterior chamber and thickened choroid and sclera but with no other anatomical malformations. Preoperative evaluation is essential for adequate surgical planning, predicting possible complications, and determining visual prognosis. Comparing the best corrected visual acuity, refractive status (hyperopia), and the degree of cataract bilaterally is essential for surgical planning.

Preoperative evaluation is an essential aspect of hypermetropia cataract patients due to the unique anatomical and refractive characteristics of these eyes. A critical aspect of preoperative evaluation in hypermetropia cataract patients is the measurement of endothelial cell density and corneal thickness. Stănilă et al. have shown that preexisting hypermetropia can modify the evolution of intraoperative and postoperative cataract surgery, leading to a loss of endothelial cells [72]. Therefore, measuring endothelial cell density and corneal thickness before and after surgery can help to identify any changes and ensure optimal outcomes. Another important aspect of preoperative evaluation in hypermetropia cataract patients is excluding certain conditions, such as glaucoma. Noted that patients with known open-angle or angle-closure glaucoma should be excluded from refractive cataract surgery, as both conditions are associated with specific refractive errors [73]. Therefore, thoroughly evaluating the patient's ocular health must ensure that preexisting conditions are appropriately managed before cataract surgery. In addition, preoperative visual acuity is essential in hypermetropia cataract patients. A meta-analysis found that the outcome of cataract surgery, evaluated as objective and subjective visual improvement, was independent of preoperative visual acuity [74]. However, preoperative patient expectations should also be considered, as cataract surgery has become well-recognized as a refractive procedure, and patient satisfaction is related to preoperative expectations [75]. In conclusion, preoperative evaluation is essential for cataract surgery in hypermetropia patients. Measuring endothelial cell density and corneal thickness, excluding certain conditions, evaluating preoperative visual acuity and expectations, examining the macula, considering subjective experiences and objective functional visual outcomes, and using a risk-based approach to medical evaluation can all contribute to successful outcomes in hypermetropia cataract surgery.

However, selecting the appropriate IOL in eyes with short axial length (AL) can be challenging. Traditional IOL measurement formulas in eyes with short AL have reduced reliability. Several technical and surgical strategies have been proposed to optimize the visual outcome and decrease the rate of surgical complications. It is essential to understand their applications in these cases [76]. To compare the accuracy of a new IOL power formula (Kane formula) with existing formulas using IOLMaster, predominantly model 3, biometry, and optimized lens constants, it found that the Kane formula was more accurate than existing formulas. Röggla et al. found that the Haigis formula showed the highest percentage of cases with ≤ 0.5 D in eyes with a short AL [77]. In eyes with short AL, the Haigis formula helps calculate IOL power length and estimate the postoperative effective lens position (ELP) using preoperative anterior chamber depth and axial length [78].

3.4.1 Cataract surgery on small eyes

As expected, cataract surgery in small eyes has inherent anatomical challenges that must be addressed to prevent complications. The most commonly reported complications are posterior capsule rupture, zonular dehiscence, iris prolapse, corneal endothelial/Descemet membrane trauma, transient severe corneal edema, cystoid macular edema (CME), severe anterior uveitis, uveal effusion, angle-closure glaucoma, retinal detachment, and aqueous misdirection [79]. These eyes also have a higher risk of severe complications during cataract surgery, including uveal effusion or suprachoroidal hemorrhage. Pressure fluctuations during the surgery should be limited to reduce the risk of these complications. Reported that using a soft-shell technique with viscoelastic agents can help maintain a stable anterior chamber and reduce the risk of complications. Iris expansion devices are commonly used to visualize the surgical field better during cataract surgery. However, these devices can cause iris trauma and increase the risk of complications in small eyes. The iris hooks are better than most iris expansion devices for small eyes. Preoperative intravenous mannitol can dehydrate the vitreous, reducing its volume and the likelihood of significant posterior pressure during cataract surgery in small eyes. It reported that intravenous mannitol can be used safely and effectively in small eyes to reduce the risk of complications. Sometimes, a vitreous tap may be necessary to reduce the risk of complications during cataract surgery in small eyes. A vitreous tap can be performed using a trocar system, which may limit complications from pars plana vitrectomy in small eyes.

Postoperative refractive error is another concern in hypermetropia cataract patients. It reported that preoperative IOL power calculation using A-scan and biometry could help achieve the desired postoperative refractive status. In addition, postoperative management should include regular follow-up visits to monitor visual acuity and potential complications. In conclusion, hypermetropic cataract patients may experience difficulties during and after surgery, including posterior capsular thickening, uveal effusion or suprachoroidal hemorrhage, inflammation, and refractive error. To manage these complications, a personalized approach should be used, taking into account the individual characteristics of each patient. Regular follow-up visits are also essential to monitor visual acuity and potential complications.

3.5 Astigmatism

Astigmatism is a standard refractive error that can cause blurred vision and decreased visual acuity. Cataract surgery allows one to correct preexisting astigmatism, improving visual outcomes, and reducing the need for glasses or contact lenses. There are several techniques for correcting preexisting astigmatism during cataract surgery. One option is corneal incisions, such as limbal relaxing incisions (LRI) or femtosecond laser-assisted astigmatic keratotomy (FSAK). These incisions are made on the steep axis of the cornea to reduce astigmatism. Reported that FSAK and toric intraocular lens (IOL) implantation were both effective in correcting astigmatism in cataract surgery patients with corneal astigmatism ranging between 0.5 D and 4.5 D. Another option for correcting astigmatism during cataract surgery is toric IOL implantation. Toric IOLs have a specific orientation that can correct astigmatism. Reported that toric IOL implantation has higher predictability than incisional methods because it is independent of corneal wound healing. The choice of technique for astigmatism correction depends on several factors, including the severity and axis of astigmatism, the patient's age and comorbidities, and the surgeon's experience and preference. They are reported that astigmatism correction during or even after cataract surgery is a safe and effective method to improve visual outcomes. It is important to note that not all astigmatism needs to be corrected. Correcting pre-surgical astigmatism should be considered separately depending on whether a patient has residual accommodation and the type of refractive surgery under consideration. In addition, accurate alignment of toric IOLs is critical for successful astigmatism correction. They reported that a three-random-point marking method using the iTrace Aberrometer could improve the accuracy of toric IOL alignment (**Figure 1**).

In conclusion, astigmatism correction during cataract surgery can improve visual outcomes and reduce the need for glasses or contact lenses. The choice of technique depends on several factors, and accurate alignment of toric IOLs is critical for successful astigmatism correction. It is essential to consider each patient's characteristics and preferences when deciding on the best approach for astigmatism correction during cataract surgery [80].

3.6 Post-refractive surgery eyes

Corneal refractive surgery, such as LASIK, PRK, or RK, can alter the corneal curvature, making IOL power calculation challenging in cataract surgery patients. Accurate IOL power calculation is crucial for achieving the desired refractive outcome

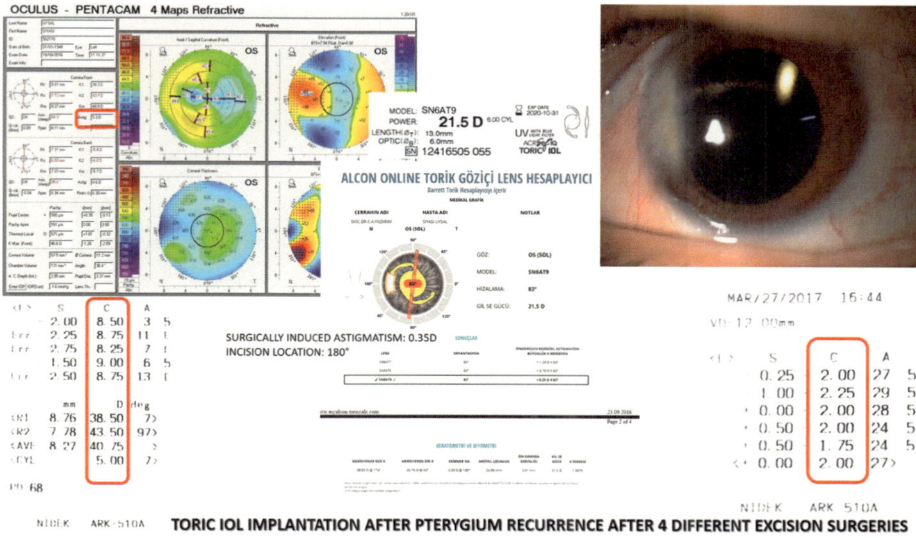

Figure 1.
Toric IOL implantation after pterygium recurrence after four different excision surgeries.

and reducing the need for additional corrective procedures. One of the main challenges in IOL power calculation after corneal refractive surgery is the altered ratio between the anterior and posterior corneal surface, which makes the keratometric index invalid. Reported that the effective lens position is erroneously predicted if such a prediction is based on the post-refractive surgery corneal curvature. Therefore, alternative methods have been proposed for measuring corneal power, such as total corneal power measurement using high-speed optical coherence tomography. Another challenge is the measurement of corneal curvature radius outside the optical zone, which can lead to an underestimation of the surgically induced refractive change. Reported that a new method, the Iida-Shimizu-Shoji (ISS) method, combines the anterior-posterior ratio of the corneal radius of curvature after LASIK to improve IOL power calculation accuracy. Several IOL power calculation formulas have been developed to address the challenges of IOL power calculation after corneal refractive surgery. The Holladay 2 formula and the American Society of Cataract and Refractive Surgery (ASCRS) Post-Refractive IOL Calculator have commonly used formulas that have been shown to provide accurate results in some studies (**Figure 2**). However, other studies have reported that IOL power calculation for eyes that have previously undergone refractive surgery is less accurate than that for virgin eyes.

The Zhang & Zheng (ZZ) formula is a newly-developed intraocular lens (IOL) calculation formula that has shown promising results in clinical accuracy analysis for post-corneal refractive surgery eyes [81]. They compared the precision of the ZZ, Haigis-L, Shammas, Barrett True-K (no history), and ray tracing (C.S.O Sirius) IOL power assessments in eyes that had undergone corneal refractive surgery. No data from before the patient's refractive procedure was used in the analysis. Compared to ray tracing, the ZZ IOL formula produced a smaller arithmetic IOL prediction error (PE; $P = 0.04$), whereas all the other formulas produced similar results ($P > 0.05$). When compared to Shammas (P 0.01), Haigis-L ($P = 0.02$), Barrett true K ($P = 0.03$), and ray tracing (P 0.01), ZZ IOL produced a lower absolute IOL PE. They theorized that the ZZ IOL formula could provide better results for calculating the power of

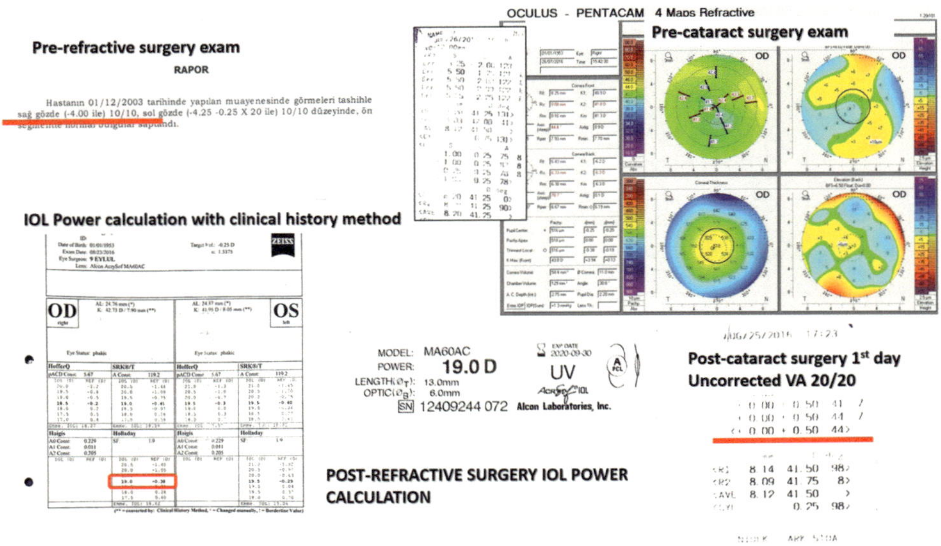

Figure 2.
Post-refractive surgery IOL power calculation.

an IOL in eyes that have undergone corneal refractive surgery but do not have any preexisting refractive data.

In addition, the type of multifocal IOL used can also affect the accuracy of IOL power calculation after corneal refractive surgery. It was reported that factors such as the type of multifocal IOL, the degree of preoperative refractive error, and the amount of corneal astigmatism could affect the prediction error after cataract surgery with implantation of various multifocal IOLs in patients with previous refractive laser surgery. In conclusion, IOL power calculation after corneal refractive surgery is challenging due to the altered corneal curvature and the invalidity of the keratometric index. Alternative methods for measuring corneal power and new IOL power calculation formulas have been developed to improve accuracy. Considering each patient's characteristics and the type of IOL used when calculating IOL power after corneal refractive surgery is essential [82].

3.7 Eyes with corneal ectasias

Cataract surgery is a standard procedure that can improve visual acuity in cataract patients. However, cataract surgery in patients with keratoconus poses particular challenges due to the altered corneal shape and thickness. Preoperative workup for cataract surgery in keratoconus patients is crucial to ensure accurate IOL power calculation and identify potential complications. Ton et al. investigated the visual and refractive outcomes in patients with keratoconus having cataract surgery with a toric IOL. They compared the IOL power calculation accuracy of conventional formulas and keratoconus-specific formulas [83]. They found that the Barrett Universal II, Holladay 2, and SRK/T were the most accurate IOL power calculation formulas in patients with keratoconus undergoing cataract surgery. Additionally, a study reported that a planned combination of primary and piggyback IOLs implantation in keratoconus at the time of cataract surgery could correct complex refractive defects associated with the disease [84]. Toric IOL implantation is a viable option for correcting astigmatism in keratoconus patients undergoing cataract surgery. Allard et al. l. reported a case of successful toric IOL implantation in a patient with keratoconus and previous penetrating keratoplasty (PKP) in one eye [85]. Additionally, some reports have been published about a two-stage surgical intervention in patients with keratoconus and cataracts to correct ametropia and prevent disease progression effectively. They initially implanted Ferrara 150–350 μm intrastromal corneal ring segments (ICRS). In Stage 2, to rectify the remaining refractive error, the hazy lens was removed and replaced with a toric posterior chamber intraocular lens (TIOL) in five to seven months [86]. The conclusion was that two-stage surgery could correct ametropia in individuals with keratoconus and cataracts.

It is important to note that cataract surgery in keratoconus patients may carry a risk of corneal ectasia following surgery. A rapidly progressive corneal ectasia was reported in a patient with keratoconus following uncomplicated phacoemulsification surgery for cataract removal [87]. Therefore, careful preoperative evaluation and postoperative monitoring are essential to minimize the risk of complications.

In conclusion, cataract surgery in keratoconus patients requires careful preoperative evaluation and planning to ensure accurate IOL power calculation and identify potential complications. Toric IOL implantation and a two-stage surgical intervention may be necessary to correct ametropia and astigmatism effectively. It is essential to consider each patient's characteristics and the potential risks and benefits when deciding on the best approach for cataract surgery in keratoconus patients.

3.8 Eyes with sequential/simultaneous vitreoretinal surgery

Cataract surgery with sequential or simultaneous vitreoretinal surgery is a complex procedure that requires careful planning and execution. The literature suggests that combined surgery is recommended for selected patients with simultaneous vitreoretinal pathological changes and cataracts [88–90]. However, the optimal timing and approach for combined surgery remain controversial. A comparative analysis of two-stage or simultaneous vitreoretinal surgery results with phacoemulsification in patients with advanced proliferative diabetic retinopathy and complicated incipient cataract showed that both approaches could be practical [91, 92]. The choice of approach may depend on the severity of the retinopathy and the degree of cataract. Patients with a history of trauma, pseudoexfoliation syndrome, degenerative myopia, uveitis, retinitis pigmentosa, and previous vitreoretinal surgery are at increased risk for complications during combined surgery [93]. Therefore, careful preoperative evaluation and planning are essential to minimize the risk of complications. Most British and Eire Association of Vitreoretinal Surgeons members would use the opposite eye biometry in a patient with a cataract and macula-off rhegmatogenous retinal detachment undergoing combined phaco-vitrectomy surgery. In contrast, most Punjab surgeons would leave the patient aphakic [94]. This highlights the importance of considering each patient's characteristics and the potential risks and benefits when deciding on the best approach for combined surgery. The level of proinflammatory cytokines in tear of patients with advanced proliferative diabetic retinopathy and complicated primary cataract after phacoemulsification surgery and IOL implantation with vitreoretinal surgery accomplished at once in comparison with vitreoretinal surgery only has been studied [95]. The results showed that combined surgery did not significantly increase the level of proinflammatory cytokines in tears. Clear corneal phacoemulsification combined with 25-gauge transconjunctival sutureless vitrectomy and standard 20-gauge vitrectomy for patients with cataracts and vitreoretinal diseases has been compared [96]. The study showed that both approaches were safe and effective, with no significant differences in visual outcomes or complication rates.

In conclusion, cataract surgery with sequential or simultaneous vitreoretinal surgery is a complex procedure that requires careful planning and execution. Combined surgery is recommended for selected patients with simultaneous vitreoretinal pathological changes and cataracts. However, the optimal timing and approach for combined surgery remain controversial, and careful preoperative evaluation and planning are essential to minimize the risk of complications.

3.9 Cataract surgery after vitrectomy

Cataract surgery after vitrectomy or phaco-vitrectomy is standard due to the high incidence of cataract formation after vitreoretinal surgery. According to Lahey et al., 75% of patients will develop visually significant cataracts within one year and 95% within two years after vitrectomy [97]. Therefore, cataract surgery is often necessary to restore visual function in these patients. Factors influencing refractive outcomes after combined phacoemulsification and pars plana vitrectomy have been studied by Jeoung et al. [98]. They found that the presence of silicone oil tamponade, preoperative axial length, and intraoperative complications were significant factors affecting refractive outcomes. In a study by Do et al., the effectiveness and safety of surgery for post-vitrectomy cataracts were evaluated [99]. The study aimed to evaluate visual acuity, quality of life, and other outcomes. The results showed that surgery for post-vitrectomy cataracts was effective and safe in improving visual acuity and quality of life. Fernandez has also studied cataract formation following pars plana vitrectomy in the pediatric population [100]. The study aimed to analyze post-vitrectomy cataract formation in the pediatric population and the perioperative factors affecting cataract development in these patients. The conclusion was that pediatric eye care providers should know the significant risk of cataract formation following phakic PPV.

In conclusion, cataract surgery after vitrectomy is expected due to the high incidence of cataract formation after vitreoretinal surgery. Factors such as silicone oil tamponade, preoperative axial length, and intraoperative complications can affect refractive outcomes. Surgery for post-vitrectomy cataracts effectively and safely improves visual acuity and quality of life.

4. Conclusions

In summary, the evolution of biometric intraocular lens calculation formulas and IOL selection in challenging cases are advancing rapidly. The development of optical biometers, surgical techniques, types of IOLs, and accurate formulas for their adequate selection has significantly improved cataract surgery outcomes over the years. The current trend in IOL selection aims to achieve optimal refractive outcomes by utilizing accurate corneal and biometric measurements, advanced formulas, and improved IOL designs. With these advancements, potential complications arise, that include incorrect lens power, optical aberrations, and IOL dislocation, which can lead to explantation. However, with the use of advanced techniques, patient selection, and appropriate biometric parameters, cataract surgery outcomes continue to improve, providing greater visual outcomes and a higher quality of life for patients.

Intraocular lens selection in challenging cases requires careful consideration of various factors. The choice of IOL will depend on the patient's individual anatomy, pathology, and visual needs. Patients with irregular corneas, such as keratoconus, require special consideration to achieve optimal visual outcomes. However, the implantation of multifocal IOLs in these patients should be avoided. Various ophthalmic pathologies and systemic comorbidities can also exacerbate complications related to IOL opacification. To achieve the best results in IOL selection, clinicians should perform a thorough preoperative evaluation of the patient and appropriately select the IOL. Different IOLs and IOL power formulas have been developed, making choosing the most appropriate lens for the patient challenging. Further research is needed to refine IOL selection in challenging cases.

Author details

Ezgi Karataş[1] and Canan Aslı Utine[2,3,4]*

1 Department of Ophthalmology, İbrahim Çeçen University Faculty of Medicine, Ağrı, Türkiye

2 Department of Ophthalmology, Dokuz Eylül University Faculty of Medicine, İzmir, Türkiye

3 İzmir Biomedicine and Genome Center, İzmir, Türkiye

4 Department of Ophthalmology, University of Naples Federico II, Napoli, Italy

*Address all correspondence to: cananutine@gmail.com

References

[1] Holladay JT. Standardizing constants for ultrasonic biometry, keratometry, and intraocular lens power calculations. Journal of Cataract and Refractive Surgery. 1997;**23**(9):1356-1370

[2] Martinez-Enriquez E, Pérez-Merino P, Durán-Poveda S, Jiménez-Alfaro I, Marcos S. Estimation of intraocular lens position from full crystalline lens geometry: Towards a new generation of intraocular lens power calculation formulas. Scientific Reports. 2018;**8**(1):1-11. Available from: https://www.nature.com/articles/s41598-018-28272-6 [Accessed: May 2, 2023]

[3] Olsen T. Calculation of intraocular lens power: A review. Acta Ophthalmologica Scandinavica. 2007;**85**(5):472-485. DOI: 10.1111/j.1600-0420.2007.00879.x

[4] Gupta A, Singh P. Intraocular Lens Power Calculation. StatPearls [Internet]; 2022. Available from: https://www.ncbi.nlm.nih.gov/books/NBK589643/ [Accessed: May 7, 2023]

[5] Retzlaff J. A new intraocular lens calculation formula. Journal-American Intra-Ocular Implant Society [Internet]. 1980;**6**(2):148-152. Available from: https://pubmed.ncbi.nlm.nih.gov/7410163/ [Accessed: May 7, 2023]

[6] Holladay JT, Musgrove KH, Prager TC, Lewis JW, Chandler TY, Ruiz RS. A three-part system for refining intraocular lens power calculations. Journal of Cataract & Refractive Surgery [Internet]. 1988;**14**(1):17-24. Available from: https://pubmed.ncbi.nlm.nih.gov/3339543/ [Accessed: May 7, 2023]

[7] Hoffer KJ. The Hoffer Q formula: A comparison of theoretic and regression formulas. Journal of Cataract & Refractive Surgery [Internet]. 1993;**19**(6):700-712. Available from: https://pubmed.ncbi.nlm.nih.gov/8271165/ [Accessed: May 7, 2023]

[8] Retzlaff JA, Sanders DR, Kraff MC. Development of the SRK/T intraocular lens implant power calculation formula. Journal of Cataract & Refractive Surgery [Internet]. 1990;16(3):333-340. Available from: https://pubmed.ncbi.nlm.nih.gov/2355321/ [Accessed: May 7, 2023]

[9] Holladay JT, Gills JP, Leidlein J, Cherchio M. Achieving emmetropia in extremely short eyes with two piggyback posterior chamber intraocular lenses. Ophthalmology [Internet]. 1996;**103**(7):1118-1123. Available from: https://pubmed.ncbi.nlm.nih.gov/8684803/ [Accessed: May 7, 2023]

[10] Darcy K, Gunn D, Tavassoli S, Sparrow J, Kane JX. Assessment of the accuracy of new and updated intraocular lens power calculation formulas in 10 930 eyes from the UK National Health Service. Journal of Cataract & Refractive Surgery [Internet]. 2020;**46**(1):2-7. Available from: https://pubmed.ncbi.nlm.nih.gov/32050225/ [Accessed: May 7, 2023]

[11] Haigis W. Intraocular lens calculation after refractive surgery for myopia: Haigis-L formula. Journal of Cataract & Refractive Surgery [Internet]. 2008;**34**(10):1658-1663. Available from: https://pubmed.ncbi.nlm.nih.gov/18812114/ [Accessed: May 8, 2023]

[12] Kuthirummal N, Vanathi M, Mukhija R, Gupta N, Meel R, Saxena R, et al. Evaluation of Barrett universal II formula for intraocular lens power calculation in Asian Indian population. Indian Journal of Ophthalmology

[Internet]. 2020;68(1):59. Available from: https://www.ncbi.nlm.nih.gov/pmc/articles/PMC6951124/ [Accessed: May 20, 2023]

[13] Shin DE, Lee H, Koh K. Comparative analysis of a presbyopia-correcting intraocular lens that combines extended depth-of-focus and bifocal profiles with a standard monofocal intraocular lens. BMC Ophthalmology. 2022;**22**(1):1-7. DOI: 10.1186/s12886-022-02516-6

[14] Iijima K, Kamiya K, Iida Y, Kasahara M, Shoji N. Predictability of combined cataract surgery and trabeculectomy using Barrett Universal II formula. PLoS One [Internet]. 2022;**17**(6). Available from: https://www.ncbi.nlm.nih.gov/pmc/articles/PMC9223616/ [Accessed: Jun 13, 2023]

[15] Pantanelli SM, Sun A, Kansara N, Smits G. Comparison of Barrett and Emmetropia verifying optical toric calculators. Clinical Ophthalmology. 2022;**16**:177-182. DOI: 10.2147/OPTH.S346925

[16] Connell BJ, Kane JX. Comparison of the Kane formula with existing formulas for intraocular lens power selection. BMJ Open Ophthalmology [Internet]. 2019;**4**(1):e000251. Available from: https://bmjophth.bmj.com/content/4/1/e000251 [Accessed: May 20, 2023]

[17] Savini G, Di Maita M, Hoffer KJ, Næser K, Schiano-Lomoriello D, Vagge A, et al. Comparison of 13 formulas for IOL power calculation with measurements from partial coherence interferometry. British Journal of Ophthalmology [Internet]. 2021;**105**(4):484-489. . Available from: https://pubmed.ncbi.nlm.nih.gov/32522789/ [Accessed: May 20, 2023]

[18] Kane JX, Connell B, Yip H, McAlister JC, Beckingsale P, Snibson GR, et al. Accuracy of intraocular lens power formulas modified for patients with keratoconus. Ophthalmology [Internet]. 2020;**127**(8):1037-1042. Available from: https://pubmed.ncbi.nlm.nih.gov/32279887/ [Accessed: May 20, 2023]

[19] Tan X, Zhang J, Zhu Y, Xu J, Qiu X, Yang G, et al. Accuracy of new generation intraocular lens calculation formulas in vitrectomized eyes. American Journal of Ophthalmology. 2020;**217**:81-90

[20] Vilaltella M, Cid-Bertomeu P, Huerva V. Accuracy of 10 IOL power calculation formulas in 100 short eyes (≤ 22 mm). International Ophthalmology [Internet]. 2023. Available from: https://www.researchgate.net/publication/369555688_Accuracy_of_10_IOL_power_calculation_formulas_in_100_short_eyes_22_mm [Accessed: May 20, 2023]

[21] Wang Y, Yang F, Lou X, Qian S, Hu B, Zhao Y, et al. Efficacy of toric intraocular lens implantation in patients older than 80 years with cataracts and corneal astigmatism. Ophthalmology and Therapy [Internet]. 2023;**12**(3). Available from: https://pubmed.ncbi.nlm.nih.gov/36856976/ [Accessed: May 20, 2023]

[22] Shammas HJ, Taroni L, Pellegrini M, Shammas MC, Jivrajka R V. Accuracy of newer intraocular lens power formulas in short and long eyes using sum-of-segments biometry. Journal of Cataract & Refractive Surgery [Internet]. 2022;**48**(10):1113-1120. Available from: https://journals.lww.com/jcrs/Fulltext/2022/10000/Accuracy_of_newer_intraocular_lens_power_formulas.4.aspx [Accessed: May 20, 2023]

[23] Chang P, Qian S, Wang Y, Li S, Yang F, Hu Y, et al. Accuracy of new-generation intraocular lens calculation

formulas in eyes with variations in predicted refraction. Graefe's Archive for Clinical and Experimental Ophthalmology. 2023;**261**(1):127-135. DOI: 10.1007/s00417-022-05748-w

[24] Li H, Ye Z, Luo Y, Li Z. Comparing the accuracy of the new-generation intraocular lens power calculation formulae in axial myopic eyes: A meta-analysis. International Ophthalmology. 2023;**43**(2):619-633. DOI: 10.1007/s10792-022-02466-4

[25] Karmiris E, Gartaganis PS, Ntravalias T, Manousakis E, Giannakis I, Chalkiadaki E. Agreement between swept-source optical biometry and Scheimpflug-based tomography in eyes with previous myopic refractive surgery. Saudi Journal of Ophthalmology [Internet]. 2022;**36**(2):229. Available from: https://www.ncbi.nlm.nih.gov/pmc/articles/PMC9535920/ [Accessed: May 20, 2023]

[26] Mena-Linares EE, Ponce-Martínez JR, Messina-Baas OM, Loya-Carrera MF, Mena-Linares EE, Ponce-Martínez JR, et al. Refractive error with the Barrett true-K No History versus Panacea formula in cataract operated patients with a history of radial keratotomy. Revista médica del Hospital General de México [Internet]. 2021;**84**(4):163-168. Available from: http://www.scielo.org.mx/scielo.php?script=sci_arttext&pid=S2524-177X2021000400163&lng=es&nrm=iso&tlng=en [Accessed: May 20, 2023]

[27] Ferreira TB, Ribeiro P, Ribeiro FJ, O'Neill JG. Comparison of methodologies using estimated or measured values of total corneal astigmatism for toric intraocular lens power calculation. Journal of Refractive Surgery [Internet]. 2017;**33**(12):794-800. Available from: https://pubmed.ncbi.nlm.nih.gov/29227506/ [Accessed: May 20, 2023]

[28] Voytsekhivskyy OV, Hoffer KJ, Savini G, Tutchenko LP, Hipólito-Fernandes D. Clinical accuracy of 18 IOL power formulas in 241 short eyes. Current Eye Research. 2021;**46**(12):1832-1843. DOI: 10.1080/02713683.2021.1933056

[29] Nemeth G, Modis L. Accuracy of the Hill-Radial Basis Function method and the Barrett Universal II formula. European Journal of Ophthalmology [Internet]. 2021;**31**(2):566-571. Available from: https://pubmed.ncbi.nlm.nih.gov/31992069/ [Accessed: May 20, 2023]

[30] Li C, Wang M, Feng R, Liang F, Liu X, He C, et al. Comparison of formula-specific factors and artificial intelligence formulas with axial length adjustments in bilateral cataract patients with long axial length. Ophthalmology and Therapy [Internet]. 2022;**11**(5):1869. Available from: https://www.ncbi.nlm.nih.gov/pmc/articles/PMC9437155/ [Accessed: May 20, 2023]

[31] Voytsekhivskyy O V., Hoffer KJ, Tutchenko L, Cooke DL, Savini G. Accuracy of 24 IOL Power Calculation Methods. J Journal of Refractive Surgery [Internet]. 2023;**39**(4):249-256. Available from: https://pubmed.ncbi.nlm.nih.gov/37040214/ [Accessed: May 20, 2023]

[32] Wendelstein J, Heath M, Riaz KM, Seiler T, Cooke DL, Langenbucher A, et al. Biometry and intraocular lens power calculation in eyes with prior laser vision correction (LVC) –A review. Klinische Monatsblätter für Augenheilkunde. 2022;**239**(08):971-981. DOI: 10.1055/a-1896-0881

[33] Langenbucher A, Szentmáry N, Cayless A, Wendelstein J, Hoffmann P. Formula constant optimisation techniques including variation of keratometer or corneal refractive index and consideration for classical and modern

IOL formulae. PLoS One. 2023;**18**(2). DOI: 10.1371/journal.pone.0282213

[34] Langenbucher A, Szentmáry N, Cayless A, Weisensee J, Fabian E, Wendelstein J, et al. Considerations on the Castrop formula for calculation of intraocular lens power. PLoS One. 2021;**16**(6). DOI: 10.1371/journal.pone.0252102

[35] Wendelstein J, Hoffmann P, Hirnschall N, Fischinger IR, Mariacher S, Wingert T, et al. Project hyperopic power prediction: Accuracy of 13 different concepts for intraocular lens calculation in short eyes. British Journal of Ophthalmology. 2022;**106**(6):795-801. DOI: 10.1136/bjophthalmol-2020-318272

[36] Kesim C, Yıldız-Taş A, Karslıoğlu MZ, Hasanreisoğlu M, Müftüoğlu O, Şahin A. The effect of anterior segment depth on the accuracy of 7 different intraocular lens calculation formulas. Turkish Journal of Ophthalmology [Internet]. 2022;**52**(4):228-236. Available from: https://pubmed.ncbi.nlm.nih.gov/36016720/ [Accessed: June 13, 2023]

[37] Vasavada V. Paradigms for pediatric cataract surgery. Asia-Pacific Journal of Ophthalmology (Philadelphia, PA) [Internet]. 2018;**7**(2):123-127. Available from: https://pubmed.ncbi.nlm.nih.gov/28971632/ [Accessed: May 20, 2023]

[38] Autrata R, Řehuřek J, Vodičková K. Visual results after primary intraocular lens implantation or contact lens correction for Aphakia in the first year of age. Ophthalmologica. 2005;**219**(2):72-79. DOI: 10.1159/000083264

[39] Sachdeva V, Katukuri S, Ali M, Kekunnaya R. Second intraocular surgery after primary pediatric cataract surgery: Indications and outcomes during long-term follow-up at a Tertiary Eye Care Center. Eye. 2016;**30**(9):1260-1265. DOI: 10.1038/eye.2016.170

[40] Lambert SR, Lynn MJ, Hartmann EE, DuBois L, Drews-Botsch C, Freedman SF, et al. Comparison of contact lens and intraocular lens correction of monocular Aphakia during infancy. JAMA Ophthalmology. 2014;**132**(6):676-682. DOI: 10.1001/jamaophthalmol.2014.531

[41] Freedman SF, Lynn MJ, Beck AD, Bothun ED, Örge FH, Lambert SR. Glaucoma-related adverse events in the first 5 years after unilateral cataract removal in the Infant Aphakia Treatment Study. JAMA Ophthalmology. 2015;**133**(8):907-914. DOI: 10.1001/jamaophthalmol.2015.1329

[42] Bothun ED, Wilson ME, Vanderveen DK, Plager DA, Freedman SF, Trivedi RH, et al. Outcomes of bilateral cataracts removed in infants 1 to 7 months of age using the toddler Aphakia and pseudophakia treatment study registry. Ophthalmology. 2020;**127**(4):501-510. DOI: 10.1016/j.ophtha.2019.10.039

[43] Bothun ED, Lynn MJ, Christiansen SP, Kruger SJ, Vanderveen DK, Neely DE, et al. Strabismus surgery outcomes in the Infant Aphakia Treatment Study (IATS) at age 5 years. Journal of American Association for Pediatric Ophthalmology and Strabismus. 2016;**20**(6):501-505. DOI: 10.1016/j.jaapos.2016.09.014

[44] Bothun ED, Cleveland J, Lynn MJ, Christiansen SP, Vanderveen DK, Neely DE, et al. One-year strabismus outcomes in the Infant Aphakia Treatment Study. Ophthalmology. 2013;**120**(6):1227-1231. DOI: 10.1016/j.ophtha.2012.11.039

[45] Penman AD, Crowder KW, Watkins WA. Contact lens versus intraocular lens correction of monocular

Aphakia during infancy. In: 50 Studies Every Ophthalmologist Should Know. 2020. pp. 297-302. DOI: 10.1093/med/9780190050726.003.0049.

[46] Vanderveen D. Cataract surgery in infants: Should I implant an IOL? Acta Ophthalmologica. 2014;**92**. DOI: 10.1111/j.1755-3768.2014.3452.x

[47] Mohan A, Sen P, Jain R, Shah C, Jain E, Sen A. Posterior optic buttonholing of intraocular lens implantation through posterior capsulorrhexis margin: A technique of intraocular lens implantation in cases of anterior capsulorrhexis extension in pediatric cataract surgery. Indian Journal of Ophthalmology. 2021;**69**(4):974-977. DOI: 10.4103/ijo.ijo_1622_20

[48] Rong X, Ji Y, Fang Y, Jiang Y, Lu Y. Long-term visual outcomes of secondary intraocular lens implantation in children with congenital cataracts. PLoS One. 2015;**10**(7). DOI: 10.1371/journal.pone.0134864

[49] Chen D, Gong XH, Xie H, Zhu XN, Li J, Zhao YE. The long-term anterior segment configuration after pediatric cataract surgery and the association with secondary glaucoma. Scientific Reports. 2017;**7**(1). DOI: 10.1038/srep43015

[50] Liu Z, Lin H, Jin G, Tan X, Qu B, Jin L, et al. In-the-bag versus ciliary sulcus secondary intraocular lens implantation for Pediatric Aphakia: A prospective comparative study. American Journal of Ophthalmology. 2022;**236**:183-192. DOI: 10.1016/j.ajo.2021.10.006

[51] Lin H, Tan X, Lin Z, Chen J, Luo L, Wu X, et al. Capsular outcomes differ with capsulorhexis sizes after pediatric cataract surgery: A randomized controlled trial. Scientific Reports. 2015;**5**(1). DOI: 10.1038/srep16227

[52] Kavitha V, Balasubramanian P, Heralgi M. Posterior iris fixated intraocular lens for pediatric traumatic cataract. Middle East African Journal of Ophthalmology. 2016;**23**(2):215-218. DOI: 10.4103/0974-9233.171777

[53] Yu YS, Kim SJ, Choung HK. Posterior chamber intraocular lens implantation in pediatric cataract with microcornea and/or microphthalmos. Korean Journal of Ophthalmology. 2006;**20**(3):151-155. DOI: 10.3341/kjo.2006.20.3.151

[54] Zou Y, Jin L, Qu B, et al. Safety and efficacy in pediatric secondary intraocular lens implantation, in-the-bag versus sulcus implantation: A multicenter, single-blinded randomized controlled trial. Trials. 2023;**24**:388. DOI: 10.1186/s13063-023-07411-z

[55] Vasavada V, Shah SK, Vasavada VA, Vasavada AR, Trivedi RH, Srivastava S, et al. Comparison of IOL power calculation formulae for pediatric eyes. Eye (London) [Internet]. 2016;**30**(9):1242-1250. Available from: https://pubmed.ncbi.nlm.nih.gov/27494083/ [Accessed: May 21, 2023]

[56] Crouch ER, Crouch ER, Pressman SH. Prospective analysis of pediatric pseudophakia: Myopic shift and postoperative outcomes. Journal of AAPOS [Internet]. 2002;**6**(5):277-282. Available from: https://pubmed.ncbi.nlm.nih.gov/12381985/ [Accessed: May 21, 2023]

[57] Astle WF, Ingram AD, Isaza GM, Echeverri P. Pediatric pseudophakia: Analysis of intraocular lens power and myopic shift. Clinical & Experimental Ophthalmology. Apr 2007;**35**(3): 244-251

[58] Ohno-Matsui K. Pathologic myopia. Asia-Pacific Journal of Ophthalmology (Philadelphia, PA)

[Internet]. 2016;5(6):415-423. Available from: https://pubmed.ncbi.nlm.nih.gov/27898445/ [Accessed: May 21, 2023]

[59] Pan CW, Boey PY, Cheng CY, Saw SM, Tay WT, Wang JJ, et al. Myopia, axial length, and age-related cataract: The Singapore Malay eye study. Investigative Ophthalmology & Visual Science [Internet]. 2013;54(7):4498-4502. Available from: https://pubmed.ncbi.nlm.nih.gov/23737473/ [Accessed: May 21, 2023]

[60] Venkateswaran N, Henderson BA. Loose zonules in cataract surgery. Current Opinion in Ophthalmology. 2022;**33**(1):53-57. DOI: 10.1097/icu.0000000000000826

[61] Kumar S, Sarwar S, Kumar R. Outcome of phacoemulsification with intraocular lens implantation in patients with high myopia. Journal of Evolution of Medical and Dental Sciences. 2015;**4**(92):15771-15774. DOI: 10.14260/jemds/2015/2279

[62] Bozkurt TK, Miller KM. Suprachoroidal hemorrhage during femtosecond laser assisted cataract surgery. American Journal of Ophthalmology Case Reports. 2016;**4**:45-46. DOI: 10.1016/j.ajoc.2016.08.010

[63] Rongrong Z, Fu L, Yan Y, Tiantian W, Changfan W. Factors affecting early postoperative visual acuity in cataract patients with high myopia. International Journal of Ophthalmology and Clinical Research. 2020;7(3). DOI: 10.23937/2378-346x/1410117

[64] Jivrajka R, Shammas MC, Boenzi T, Swearingen M, Shammas HJ. Variability of axial length, anterior chamber depth, and lens thickness in the cataractous eye. Journal of Cataract and Refractive Surgery. 2008;**34**(2):289-294. DOI: 10.1016/j.jcrs.2007.10.015

[65] Jeon H, Jang JH, Kwon S. Risk factors for early and late intraocular lens dislocation. Journal of the Korean Ophthalmological Society. 2023;**64**(2):114-122. DOI: 10.3341/jkos.2023.64.2.114

[66] Wang H, Ramjiani V, Auger G, Raynor M, Currie Z, Tan J. Practice of immediate sequential bilateral cataract surgery (ISBCS): A teaching hospital experience in United Kingdom. European Journal of Ophthalmology. 3 Feb 2023:11206721231154609. DOI: 10.1177/11206721231154609. PMID: 36734082 [Epub ahead of print]

[67] Tan Y, Liu L, Li J, Qin Y, Sun A, Wu M. Evaluation of preoperative corneal astigmatism using swept-source optical biometry in Chinese cataract surgery candidates with high myopia: A prospective, comparative observational study. Annals of Translational Medicine. 2021;**9**(8):618-618. DOI: 10.21037/atm-20-6757

[68] Zhang M, Qian D, Jing Q, Chen J, Jiang Y. Analysis of corneal spherical aberrations in cataract patients with high myopia. Scientific Reports. 2019;**9**(1). DOI: 10.1038/s41598-018-36539-1

[69] Micovic S, Perova A. The experience of using negative power IOLs for a cataract complicated by extremely high myopia. Modern Technologies in Ophtalmology. 2021;**2**:60-62. DOI: 10.25276/2312-4911-2021-2-60-62

[70] Odenthal MTP, Eggink CA, Melles G, Pameyer JH, Geerards AJM, Houdijn BW. Clinical and theoretical results of intraocular lens power calculation for cataract surgery after photorefractive keratectomy for myopia. Archives of Ophthalmology. 2002;**120**(4):431-438. DOI: 10.1001/archopht.120.4.431

[71] Ang RT, Rapista AB, Remo JM, Tan-Daclan MT, Cruz E. Clinical

outcomes and comparison of intraocular lens calculation formulas in eyes with long axial myopia. Taiwan Journal of Ophthalmology. 2022;**12**(3):305. DOI: 10.4103/tjo.tjo_7_21

[72] Stanila DM, Florea AM, Stănilă A, Panga AA. Endothelial cells loss to the hyperopic pacients during phacoemulsification. Romanian Journal of Ophthalmology. 2017;**61**(4):256-260. DOI: 10.22336/rjo.2017.46

[73] Perkins ES. Cataract: Refractive error, diabetes, and morphology. British Journal of Ophthalmology. 1984;**68**(5):293-297. DOI: 10.1136/bjo.68.5.293

[74] Kessel L, Andresen J, Erngaard D, Flesner P, Tendal B, Hjortdal J. Indication for cataract surgery. Do we have evidence of who will benefit from surgery? A systematic review and meta-analysis. Acta Ophthalmologica. 2016;**94**(1):10-20. DOI: 10.1111/aos.12758

[75] Hawker MJ, Madge SN, Baddeley PA, Perry SR. Refractive expectations of patients having cataract surgery. Journal of Cataract and Refractive Surgery. 2005;**31**(10):1970-1975. DOI: 10.1016/j.jcrs.2005.03.065

[76] Elhusseiny AM, Sallam AB. Cataract surgery in adult eyes with short axial length. Current Opinion in Ophthalmology. 2023;**34**(1):84-93. DOI: 10.1097/icu.0000000000000913

[77] Röggla V, Langenbucher A, Leydolt C, Schartmüller D, Schwarzenbacher L, Abela-Formanek C, et al. Accuracy of common IOL power formulas in 611 eyes based on axial length and corneal power ranges. British Journal of Ophthalmology. 2021;**105**(12):1661-1665. DOI: 10.1136/bjophthalmol-2020-315882

[78] Kumar HM, Sangeetha T, Kanthamani BNJ. Comparison of accuracy of haigis and SRK II formula for intraocular lens power calculation in eyes with short axial length. Indian Journal of Clinical and Experimental Ophthalmology. 2019;**5**(3):376-381. DOI: 10.18231/j.ijceo.2019.090

[79] Cataract Surgery in Small Eyes-EyeWiki [Internet]. Available from: https://eyewiki.aao.org/Cataract_Surgery_in_Small_Eyes [Accessed: May 21, 2023]

[80] Noh H, Yoo YS, Shin KY, Lim DH, Chung TY. Comparison of penetrating femtosecond laser-assisted astigmatic keratotomy and toric intraocular lens implantation for correction of astigmatism in cataract surgery. Scientific Reports. 2021;**11**(1). DOI: 10.1038/s41598-021-86763-5

[81] Zhang J, Shao J, Zheng L, Shen Y, Zhao X. Comparative clinical accuracy analysis of the newly developed ZZ IOL and four existing IOL formulas for post-corneal refractive surgery eyes. BMC Ophthalmology. 2021;**21**(1):1-9. DOI: 10.1186/s12886-021-01991-7

[82] Patel RH, Karp CL, Yoo SH, Amescua G, Galor A. Cataract surgery after refractive surgery. International Ophthalmology Clinics [Internet]. 2016;**56**(2):171. Available from: https://www.ncbi.nlm.nih.gov/pmc/articles/PMC4780227/ [Accessed: May 21, 2023]

[83] Ton Y, Barrett GD, Kleinmann G, Levy A, Assia EI. Toric intraocular lens power calculation in cataract patients with keratoconus. Journal of Cataract & Refractive Surgery [Internet]. 2021;**47**(11):1389-1397. Available from: https://pubmed.ncbi.nlm.nih.gov/33770295/ [Accessed: June 13, 2023]

[84] Franco FGS, Nicolosi C, Vicini G, Grasso Cannizzo P, Virgili G, Giansanti F. Combining primary and

sulcus piggyback IOLs for the correction of a spherical-cylindrical defect in an eye with abnormal cornea. European Journal of Ophthalmology. 2023;**33**(1):NP64-NP68. DOI: 10.1177/11206721211037824

[85] Allard K, Zetterberg M. Toric IOL implantation in a patient with keratoconus and previous penetrating keratoplasty: A case report and review of literature. BMC Ophthalmology. 2018;**18**(1). DOI: 10.1186/s12886-018-0895-y

[86] Bikbov MM, Orenburkina OI, Babushkin AE, Nuriev IF. Two-stage treatment of ametropia in patients with keratoconus and cataracts. Acta Biomedica Scientifica. 2021;**6**(6-1):204-213. DOI: 10.29413/abs.2021-6.6-1.23

[87] Labiris G, Panagiotopoulou EK, Ntonti P, Taliantzis S. Corneal ectasia following cataract extraction surgery in a patient with keratoconus: A case report. Journal of Medical Case Reports. 2019;**13**(1). DOI: 10.1186/s13256-019-2238-x

[88] Jun Z, Pavlovic S, Jacobi KW. Results of combined vitreoretinal surgery and phacoemulsification with intraocular lens implantation. Clinical & Experimental Ophthalmology. 2001;**29**(5):307-311. DOI: 10.1046/j.1442-9071.2001.00439.x

[89] Li W, Sun G, Wu R, Wang X, Xu M, Sun C. Longterm results after phacovitrectomy and foldable intraocular lens implantation. Acta Ophthalmologica. 2009;**87**(8):896-900. DOI: 10.1111/j.1755-3768.2008.01383.x

[90] Wensheng L, Wu R, Wang X, Xu M, Sun G, Sun C. Clinical complications of combined phacoemulsification and vitrectomy for eyes with coexisting cataract and vitreoretinal diseases. European Journal of Ophthalmology. 2009;**19**(1):37-45. DOI: 10.1177/112067210901900106

[91] Konovalova K, Игоревна КК, Shishkin MA, Михайлович ШИ. Two-stage or single-stage vitreoretinal surgery with phacoemulsification in patients with advanced proliferative diabetic retinopathy? Ophthalmology Reports. 2020;**12**(4):43-48. DOI: 10.17816/ov16065

[92] Konovalova KI, Shishkin MM. Comparative evaluation of the results of simultaneous and two-stage surgical treatment of patients with advanced proliferative diabetic retinopathy and complicated incipient cataract. Modern Technologies in Ophtalmology. 2021;**2**:38-42. DOI: 10.25276/2312-4911-2021-2-38-42

[93] Patel SN, Snyder LL. Reverse suture technique for intraocular lens refixation. Retinal Cases & Brief Reports. 2021;**15**(5):625-627. DOI: 10.1097/icb.0000000000000867

[94] Brent AJ, Bedi S, Wakefield M, Banerjee S. A comparative study of lens management in the United Kingdom and India with regard to rhegmatogenous retinal detachment surgery. European Journal of Ophthalmology. 2020;**30**(5):1120-1126. DOI: 10.1177/1120672119855209

[95] Konovalova KI, Shishkin MM, Fayzrakhmanov RR. Comparative analysis of the level of proinflammatory cytokines in tear of patients with advanced proliferative diabetic retinopathy and complicated primary cataract. Modern Technologies in Ophtalmology. 2022;**1**:61-66. DOI: 10.25276/2312-4911-2022-1-61-66

[96] Chang CJ, Chang YH, Chiang SY, Lin LT. Comparison of clear corneal phacoemulsification combined with

25-gauge transconjunctival sutureless vitrectomy and standard 20-gauge vitrectomy for patients with cataract and vitreoretinal diseases. Journal of Cataract and Refractive Surgery. 2005;**31**(6):1198-1207. DOI: 10.1016/j.jcrs.2004.11.041

[97] Lahey JM, Francis RR, Fong DS, Kearney JJ, Tanaka S. Combining phacoemulsification with vitrectomy for treatment of macular holes. British Journal of Ophthalmology. 2002;**86**(8):876-878. DOI: 10.1136/bjo.86.8.876

[98] Jeoung JW, Chung H, Yu HG. Factors influencing refractive outcomes after combined phacoemulsification and pars plana vitrectomy. Journal of Cataract and Refractive Surgery. 2007;**33**(1):108-114. DOI: 10.1016/j.jcrs.2006.09.017

[99] Do DV, Gichuhi S, Vedula SS, Hawkins BS. Surgery for post-vitrectomy cataract. Cochrane Database of Systematic Reviews. 2013;**2013**(12). DOI: 10.1002/14651858.cd006366.pub3

[100] Fernandez TA, Carr EW, Hajrasouliha AR. Cataract formation following pars plana vitrectomy in the pediatric population. Journal of Pediatric Ophthalmology and Strabismus. 21 Feb 2023:1-6

Chapter 5

Cataract Surgery Complications: *Vitreo-Retina Perspectives*

Mohamed Al-Abri, Washoo Mal and Nawal Al-Fadhil

Abstract

Cataract surgery is one of the most common and successful intraocular surgeries performed worldwide. However, sight-threatening complications that involve the posterior segment can occur. The incidence of such complications is relatively low, but it is important to recognize these complications early and treat them appropriately. In this chapter, we will address some of the important posterior segment complications of cataract surgery such as intraoperative complications (e.g., vitreous loss, retained lens matter, and suprachoroidal hemorrhage) and short- and long-term postoperative complications (e.g., postoperative endophthalmitis, rhegmatogenous retinal detachment, cystoid macular edema and progression of preexisting diabetic retinopathy, and/or diabetic macular edema).

Keywords: cataract surgery, complications, posterior segment, retina, vitreous, diabetic retinopathy, diabetic macular edema

1. Introduction

Cataract surgery is one of the most common and successful intraocular surgeries performed worldwide. With latest innovations and technologies, such a surgery became easy to perform with less operating time and shorter postoperative recovery period. However, sight-threatening complications that involve the posterior segment can occur. The incidence of such complications is relatively low, but it is important to recognize these complications early and treat them appropriately. In this chapter, we will address some of the important posterior segment complications of cataract surgery such as intraoperative complications (e.g., vitreous loss, retained lens matter, and suprachoroidal hemorrhage) and short- and long-term postoperative complications (e.g., postoperative endophthalmitis, rhegmatogenous retinal detachment, cystoid macular edema and progression of preexisting diabetic retinopathy, and/or diabetic macular edema).

2. Vitreous loss and retained lens matter

An intact posterior lens capsule (PC) is an important normal anatomical barrier, which separates the vitreous body from the forces resulting from cataract surgery and intraocular lens (IOL) implantation. The incidence of PC tear and vitreous loss is variable depending on the surgeon's skills, years of experience, surgical volume, and complexity of cataract case mix.

The reported incidence ranges from 0.45–8.22% [1–3].

Vitreous loss can lead to an increased risk of sight-threatening complications, including cystoid macular edema, retinal detachment, and endophthalmitis [4–6]. Significant PC tear might be followed by dislocation of lens fragment(s) into the vitreous cavity [7].

Prevention: Risk stratification is an important measure to reduce such risk by appropriate patient selection, pre-op preparation (for detailed counseling, selecting the appropriate type of anesthesia as well as time of posting the case, and selection of surgeon experienced in dealing with complex cataract surgery).

Intra-operatively, recognizing signs of PC tear and vitreous loss are crucial. The signs to observe are sudden deepening of the anterior chamber (AC), excess sideways shift of the nucleus, sudden appearance of a red reflex, and abnormal movement of the pupillary margin distant from instruments in the AC secondary to traction transmitted through vitreous strands. If any of above signs were observed, viscodispersive substance was to be injected immediately into the AC directly above the site of PC tear while the irrigation is on to minimize vitreous prolapse and to stabilize any remaining lens fragments. At this point, the surgeon should assess the situation and change the approach appropriately for such a challenge, for example, setting up anterior vitrectomy and augmenting the local anesthesia if needed. The ultimate goals of management of PC tear and vitreous loss are removal of the prolapsed vitreous from the AC and surgical wounds, safe removal of the remaining lens fragment(s), and safe IOL implantation. The prolapsed vitreous should be removed with anterior vitrectomy with highest cut rate provided by the machine and maintaining stable AC and IOP. A sutureless vitrectomy technique *via* 23G pars plana anterior vitrectomy whenever appropriately possible might be the most controlled way to carry out safe

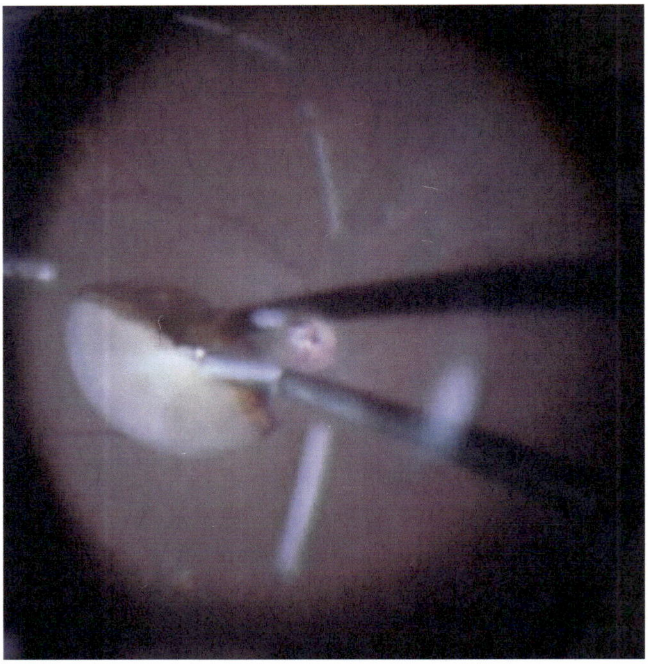

Figure 1.
Intraoperative fundus photo shows retained nuclear fragment being fragmented and removed using 23G vitrectomy probe (courtesy of Dr. M. Al-Abri).

and adequate anterior vitrectomy. This approach can be done with either an anterior chamber or pars plana infusion [8]. Such an approach mitigates AC manipulation, less risk for vitreous incarceration in the surgical wounds, and serves as logical way for adequate and safe removal of vitreous behind the plane of PC, which may preserve the residual PC from further damage. In addition, if the lens fragments threatened to fall posteriorly, pars plana approach may help in pushing the lens fragments into the AC using the vitrector. Residual soft lens matter or cortex can be safely removed using the vitrector itself. However, residual nuclear fragments can be removed either by carefully using the phaco probe, after the AC has been adequately cleaned from vitreous, or can be removed manually through an enlarged main wound. Viscoelastic or a lens glide may help to stabilize nuclear fragments in the AC before removal [9]. If appropriate, insertion of the appropriate IOL is to be done in a suitable position based on the judgment and experience of the primary surgeon. If nuclear fragments are moved posteriorly behind the plane of the PC, aggressive efforts to retrieve these fragments without pars plana vitrectomy can result in giant retinal tears and retinal detachments [10, 11]. In such cases, an urgent referral is to be made to a vitreo-retina surgeon, who can then make the appropriate decisions about the timing of the management meanwhile the patients should be monitored closely for post-op inflammation, corneal edema and IOP, and other potential complications (**Figure 1**).

3. Suprachoroidal hemorrhage

Suprachoroidal hemorrhage (SCH) is one the rare but potentially vision-threatening intraoperative or postoperative complication. It is caused by acute hypotony leading to rupture of long and short ciliary arteries, which bleed into suprachoroidal space. The incidence is extremely low, 0.03–0.81% [12].

Predisposing factors: Advanced age, uncontrolled hypertension, using anticoagulant or antiplatelet, atherosclerosis, diabetes, uncontrolled glaucoma, high axial myopia, aphakia, choroidal hemangioma, retrobulbar anesthesia, Valsalva maneuvers, and prolonged or complicated cataract surgery with vitreous loss and hypotony. Proper preoperative evaluation, identification, and management of avoidable risk factors, for example, control of high BP, high IOP, discontinue anticoagulant or antiplatelet, choose the appropriate method of anesthesia, and address cardiovascular and other systemic issues.

Clinical features: Intraoperative, progressive anterior chamber shallowing, loss of red reflex, increasing IOP with firming of eyeball, iris prolapse, vitreous extrusion, and extrusion of intraocular contents.

Intraoperative management: Terminate the surgery immediately. Gently reposition the expelled contents and quickly close the surgical wounds. Reform anterior chamber either with viscoelastic or air bubble. Immediate drainage and posterior sclerotomy are controversial.

Postoperative management: Intraocular pressure (IOP) and inflammation are controlled with IOP lowering agents (Topical Beta blocker & Carbonic anhydrase inhibitors – CAIs and/or systemic acetazolamide) and topical steroids. Cycloplegics and analgesics relieve the eye pain. NSAIDS and antiplatelets are to be avoided. Serial Ultrasound B – scan to be performed to monitor the progress and liquefaction of suprachoroidal hemorrhage (**Figure 2**).

Drainage is considered if hemorrhage does not resolve spontaneously after 2 weeks. Optimum IOP and sufficient liquefaction of clot are essential for successful

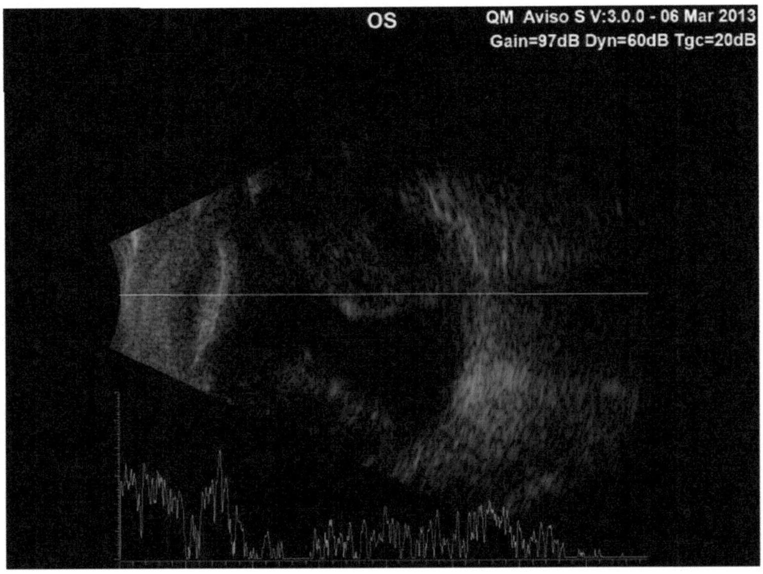

Figure 2.
B-scan ultrasound image of a patient with suprachoroidal hemorrhage post-cataract surgery. Notice the dome-shaped appearance and central apposition of detached choroid. The suprachoroidal space is filled with moderate amplitude spikes suggestive of suprachoroidal hemorrhage (courtesy of Dr. A. Al-Hinai).

procedure. The suprachoroidal lysed hemorrhage is drained either through direct 3-4 mm radial sclerotomies or transconjunctival trocar. Pars plana vitrectomy (PPV) is considered if it is complicated by retinal detachment and/or vitreous hemorrhage. Overall, visual outcome is variable and depends on the extent of SCH, associated retinal detachment as well as other ocular comorbidities. Generally, it carries poor visual prognosis especially if it is associated with retinal detachment, where some reported cases end up with <20/200 – no light perception visual acuity [13, 14].

4. Endophthalmitis post cataract surgery

Endophthalmitis is defined as intraocular inflammation involving the anterior and posterior segments of eye that could be acute, chronic or delayed onset, infective or noninfective, and exogenous or endogenous.

Acute postoperative endophthalmitis: Acute infectious endophthalmitis is a highly catastrophic and sight-threatening rare complication of cataract surgery. Presented within 6 weeks, mostly in 3–5 days with fulminant or acute course. Classic presentation is eyelid swelling, ocular pain, ciliary congestion, and sudden drop of vision, which may be associated with corneal edema, hypopyon, loss of red pupillary reflex, and purulent vitritis. (**Figure 3**).

Incidence: The incidence of acute infectious post-cataract endophthalmitis is inconsistent and varies, 0.04–0.092% [15, 16]. According to scientific literature, the incidence is globally declined with off-label (No FDA approval) use of intracameral antibiotic injections [17, 18].

Source of infection and risk factors: The flora from eyelids, conjunctiva, nasolacrimal, and infected anophthalmic socket are major sources and perioperative surgical wound contamination through a contaminated instrument or theater personnel.

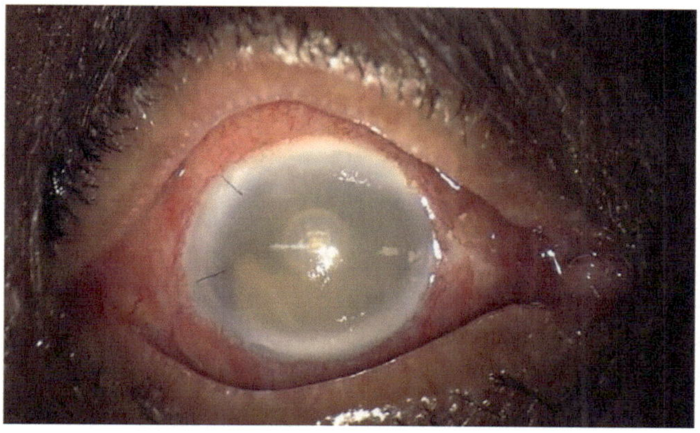

Figure 3.
Anterior segment photo of the right eye with acute endophthalmitis post-cataract surgery. Notice the diffuse conjunctival congestion, marked corneal edema, organized hypopyon, and loss of red pupillary reflex (courtesy of Dr. M. Al-Abri).

While elderly patients and immune-compromised due to diabetes mellitus, systemic malignancy, and HIV are risk factors for endogenous endophthalmitis. Other complicated surgery associated with posterior capsule rupture, vitreous loss, anterior chamber IOL, prolonged surgery, and wound leak.

Pathogens and pathogenesis: Postoperative endophthalmitis is predominantly caused by bacteria. Gram-positive isolates in almost 85% of cases. Most commonly coagulase-negative - the normal bacterial flora from eyelids. Mostly *Staphylococcus epidermidis* in 30.3%, and others are Streptococcus viridans and *Staphylococcus aureus*. The Gram-negative accounts for 10.3% (*Pseudomonas aeruginosa*, Klebsiella pneumonia) and fungi for 4.6%, including *Candida albicans* and *Aspergillus* species [19].

Once microbes get access into the eye, initiate to release intravitreal inflammatory cytokines, like tumor necrosis factor-alpha, interleukin-1 beta, and interferon-gamma that result in neutrophil migration and aggregation leading to moderate-severe suppurative inflammation and retinal tissue necrosis.

Prevention and prophylaxis: Strict aseptic measures throughout surgical process are key to infection prevention. Meticulous cleaning of periocular skin, and eyelids with 10% Povidone-Iodine solution and instillation of few drops of 5% povidone-iodine antiseptic into conjunctival cul de sac and left for 3–5 minutes followed by irrigation with sterile normal saline significantly reduce the risk of infection from adnexal flora. Proper sterile draping of surgical site with complete covering of eyelid margins and eyelashes is considered standard care. Currently, preoperative use of topical antibiotics and intracameral cefuroxime (1 mg/0.1 ml) injection at the end of surgery is common in practice [20]. Immediate closure of postoperative surgical wound leak, if noticed, is recommended.

Differential diagnosis: Post-cataract endophthalmitis must be differentiated from toxic anterior segment syndrome [TASS], keratitis, postoperative uveitis (e.g., related to retained lens material), and vitreous hemorrhage.

Management: When any suspicious postoperative endophthalmitis makes a prompt arrangement to collect specimen from aqueous with 30-G tuberculin syringe (0.1–0.2 ml) and vitreous with 23–25-G syringe (0.2–0.4 ml) to detect the causative organisms. Prepare smear for staining of Gram, Giemsa, potassium hydroxide [KOH], and culture – blood and chocolate agar, Sabouraud. Modern technology of

DNA sequencing and polymerase chain reaction (PCR) testing of vitreous biopsy is rapid and highly specific and sensitive in microbe detection but still uncommon in practice [21, 22]. Ultrasound B-scan is routinely performed to assess the severity of vitreous activity and to exclude retinal detachment.

Treatment: The intravitreal antibiotics are mainstay of treatment if visual acuity is better than light perception. Intravitreal administration of antibiotics maintains the adequate minimum inhibitory concentration (MIC) for sufficient time. The initial empirical and standard therapy is intravitreal vancomycin (1 mg/0.1 ml) for Gram-positive and ceftazidime (2.25 mg/0.1 ml) for Gram-negative bacterial coverage [23]. Ceftazidime has much better safety profile than amikacin (0.4 mg/0.1 ml), which can be used if patient is allergic to cephalosporin.

Dexamethasone (0.4 mg/0.1 ml) to halt the inflammation is an option (provided no fungal infection), however, its use is controversial because of no impact on final visual outcome. Adjuvant-fortified topical vancomycin and ceftazidime are used to address contaminated surgical wound and anterior segment involvement. Atropine 1% eye drops as cycloplegic agent is used to relieve ciliary spasm and eye pain. Systemic antibiotics are often administered.

If fungal infection is suspected or detected, intravitreal amphotericin B (5 mcg/0.1 ml) or voriconazole (100 mcg/0.1 ml) are considered. Practicing ophthalmologists are still following Endophthalmitis Vitrectomy Study (EVS) guidelines which state that pars plana vitrectomy (PPV) with intravitreal vancomycin and ceftazidime is recommended if visual acuity is only light perception [24]. However, the current practice has shifted from the EVS recommendations and recommends early PPV in hand motion or better [25, 26]. Moreover, PPV is preferred if the condition clinically worsens within 48 hours of intravitreal antibiotics rather repeat IVT injection and rarely for globe salvage in no light perception [27].

Outcomes: Overall, outcome of endophthalmitis is poor. However, outcome depends on onset, microbial virulence, and duration of the infection. Poor vision at presentation, fulminant onset, hypopyon >1.5 mm, invisible fundus and retinal detachment often have poor prognosis.

EVS describes if visual acuity is light perception at presentation (33% achieve 20/40, 56% gain 20/100 or better, and 5/200 or worse in 20% of patients [24]. Gram-negative organism-*P. aeruginosa,* Klebsiella, and infection with Bacillus species (e.g., cereus) have aggressive course and end up with severe visual loss [28].

Delayed postoperative endophthalmitis: Delayed postoperative endophthalmitis develops after 6 weeks to years of cataract surgery, and often masquerades as autoimmune uveitis. Delayed endophthalmitis has indolent course, caused by low-virulent pathogen—*Propionibacterium acnes* or *S. epidermidis*, sometimes *Aspergillus* or Candida fungi [29].

Clinical features: Painless progressive decreased visual acuity, low-grade chronic granulomatous uveitis associated with large keratic precipitates, +/− hypopyon, plaque-like material on the posterior capsule, and vitritis.

Treatment: Aqueous and vitreous specimen for staining and culture/sensitivity of microbes includes anaerobes.

Injecting antibiotics into the capsular bag or vitreous cavity usually does not eliminate the infection. Pars plana vitrectomy with complete or partial removal of capsular beg and exchange of the intraocular lens followed by intravitreal vancomycin plus ceftazidime. It is advisable to send the explanted lens and capsular beg for cultures.

Toxic anterior segment syndrome (TASS): TASS is an acute postoperative anterior chamber sterile inflammatory reaction. Noninfectious material, such as contaminants from surgical equipment, viscoelastic, intraocular lens implant, or solution toxins, enters the anterior segment and develops toxic reaction to the intraocular structure within 12–24 hours after uneventful cataract surgery.

Clinical features: Decreased visual acuity, mild or no eye pain, limbus to limbus corneal edema, moderate-severe anterior chamber reaction with cells, flares, sterile hypopyon and fibrin, and pupil may be dilated and sluggish to nonreactive and +/− high intraocular pressure.

Treatment: It responds very well to intensive topical steroid q1 hourly (e.g., prednisolone 1%), and cycloplegic (e.g., cyclopentolate 1%) with IOP monitoring.

5. Pseudophakic rhegmatogenous retinal detachment

Cataract surgery is one of the most commonly performed intraocular surgery with this there is increased interest in the potential postoperative pseudophakic rhegmatogenous retinal detachment (PRD) (**Figure 4**).

PRD is an uncommon complication after cataract surgery; the reported incidence varies widely within a range of 0.16 to 3.55% and an average of 0.7% [30–32], which is higher than in the general population (incidence of 0.0063–0.0179%) [33, 34]. Most of the reported PRD occurs within 1–2 years of the cataract removal. In a large cohort Korean study, it was found that 80% of PRD occurred within 1 year after cataract surgery [35] and another study from Moorfield's Eye Hospital found that 75% of PRD occurred within the first 2 postoperative years [36]. However, others found that the mean time between cataract surgery to PRD diagnosis was 40 months and even after 4 years [37].

Risk factors: Myopia is a well-known risk factor for PRD with 4.2- to 6.1-fold increased risk of PRD in high myopia and 1.6 to 3.2 in moderate myopia [31, 38–40]. Therefore, peripheral retinal degeneration changes predisposing to retinal detachment are commonly found in myopic eyes to be thoroughly evaluated and treated

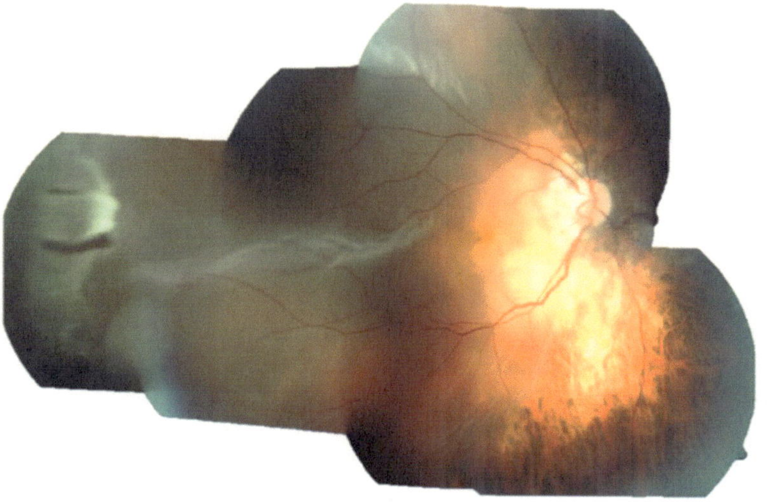

Figure 4.
Right eye fundus photo of a 27-year-old male status post ICL implantation for high myopia (AL 31.06) showing myopic fundus, macula-off retinal detachment with HST at 9 o'clock position (courtesy of Dr. M. Al-Abri).

prophylactically at least 2 weeks prior to performing cataract surgery. It has been suggested that younger age had a linear relationship with risk of PRD [40]. In a Korean population-based study, the estimated 5-year risk of RD was inversely correlated with the mean age of the patients (4.26, 2.38, 0.94, and 0.43% for patients of age groups 40–54, 55–64, 65–74, and ≥ 75, respectively; $p < 0.0001$) [35].

The increased risk of PRD in young population could be attributed to various etiologies; cataract surgery itself may induce posterior vitreous detachment (PVD), which may lead to retinal breaks, leading to RD [41, 42]. Another explanation is that the underlying causes for cataract formation in younger age group might act as predisposing factors for PRD. For example, the effect of unreported and under-detected eye trauma or myopia may be misinterpreted as the effect of younger age. In recent years, relatively early cataract surgery with multifocal IOL implantation is being performed as a treatment for presbyopia or clear lens exchange in even younger age groups for refractive errors. Considering the higher incidence of RD after lens extraction surgery in younger population, it is important to determine if cataract surgery is medically indicated and to have thorough discussion with patient about the risk of retinal detachment. Previous studies have reported male gender is a risk factor for the development of PRD. The cumulative 6-year RD rates were 1.90% in the male and 0.56% in the female subgroups of the prospective cohort study done in Taiwan [43]. This could be due to the possibility that men may have more history of under-reported trauma. The integrity of the posterior capsule is an important determinant of the onset of PVD and, hence, the risk of RD. The anterior movement of the vitreous, persistent anterior traction on the vitreous base due to vitreous adherence to the wound, IOL, and anterior segment structures may result in an increased risk of traction-induced peripheral retinal tears [35]. According to many studies, posterior capsular rupture (PCR) is a major risk factor for PRD [31, 38, 44]. It increases the risk of RD by 10-fold in one study [45] and in another report, an association was confirmed between PCR and RD occurrence with an odds ratio of 19.9 (95% CI 10.8–36.7) [40].

6. Cystoid macular edema

Cystoid macular edema (CME) following cataract surgery, also known as Irvine-Gass syndrome, is a common cause of visual impairment following cataract surgery, with or without intraocular lens implant. It was first reported in 1953, by A. Ray Irvine J, and then enlightened with use of fluorescence angiography by J Donald M. Gass, in 1969 [46].

Pathogenesis: There are numerous factors involved in the pathophysiology of CME. These factors include inflammation, vitreous traction, vascular instability, and light toxicity. Of all these factors, inflammation appears to be the core. Surgical manipulation triggers intracellular inflammation and releases inflammatory mediators such as prostaglandins; cytokines diffuse posteriorly into the vitreous causes breaking down the blood-aqueous and blood-retinal barriers, which leads to increased vascular permeability, accumulation of transudates in outer plexiform layer, inner nuclear layer of the retina, and microcysts coalesce to form a larger intraretinal cyst [47].

Incidence: Although CME following cataract surgery is documented to be the cause of decreased vision following surgery, the incidence of CME remains variable [48]. It is highly dependent on diagnostic criteria; earlier studies are either based on clinical findings with visual impairment or based on fluorescein angiography. However, recent research is more dependent on optical coherence tomography (OCT). Based on OCT findings, CME occurs in up to 50% of patients at 4–8 weeks postoperatively and is found in less than 3% of patients based on clinical findings along with visual impairment [48, 49].

Diagnosis*:* OCT is superior in looking at the retinal morphology and macular thickness. The test is noninvasive and can be repeated at any time, which is helpful in monitoring patients' response to treatment [50–52]. Fluorescein angiography (FA) is semi-invasive procedure, helpful to roll out other associated causes of CME for example diabetic retinopathy (DR) and retinal vein occlusion. Findings of FA include perifoveal capillary leakage giving the classic "petaloid" appearance and/or capillary dropout. Optical coherence tomography angiography (OCTA) is a noninvasive imaging modality that helps to visualize retinal vasculature and evaluation in retina perfusion [53] (**Figure** 5).

Risk factors: The predisposing risk factors include intraoperative complications (e.g., posterior capsule rupture, vitreous loss, iris trauma, and vitreous traction at the wound), previous surgical procedures (e.g., PPV and penetrating keratoplasty), preexisting ocular conditions (e.g., epiretinal membrane, retinal vein occlusion,

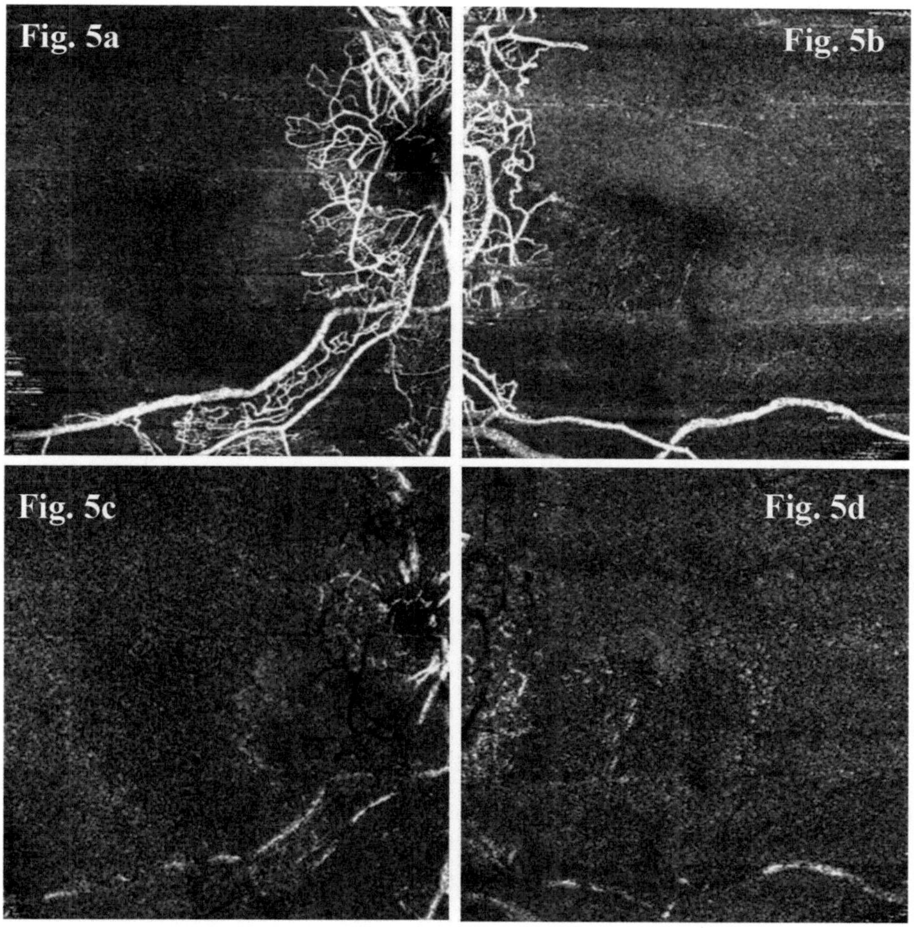

Figure 5.
Macula OCTA showing profound macular capillary dropout in both the superficial (a,b) and deep (c,d) retinal capillary plexus in both eyes (courtesy of Dr. M. Al-Abri).

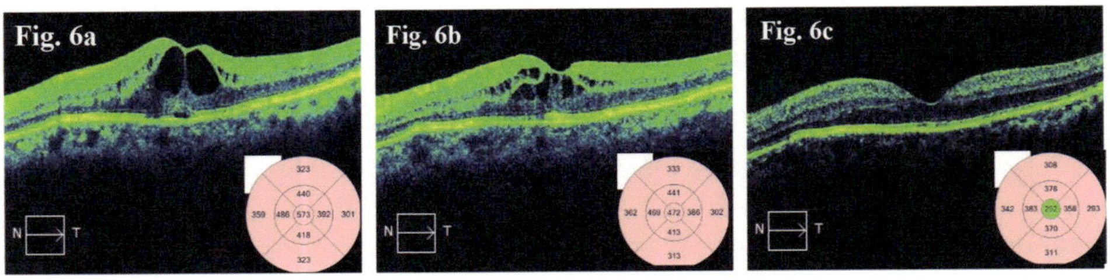

Figure 6.
OCT of the left eye with CME 4-week post-cataract surgery [BCVA 0.3] (a) and follow-up OCTs showing improvement of CME after treatment with topical nepafenac 0.1% TID for 3 and 6 months [BCVA 0.5] (c,d) (courtesy of Dr. M. Al-Abri).

uveitis, ocular hypertension and use of prostaglandin, and dry ARM), and systemic comorbidities (e.g., diabetic mellitus, hypertension, and hyperlipidemia) [54–57].

Management: CME following cataract surgery is self-limiting, where spontaneous resolution occurs within 3–6 months. Therefore, three-month observation period is recommended [56].

Although there is no high level of evidence-based guidelines for the treatment of CME following cataract surgery, most surgeons prefer to start with prophylactic topical non-steroidal antiinflammatory drugs (NSAIDs) combined with corticosteroid drops for high-risk patients [57].

NSAIDs are usually administered topically for 3–4 months and on a needed basis [58]. Previous studies concluded that a combination therapy of topical NSAIDs with corticosteroid drops is more effective than monotherapy post-operative period [59] (**Figure 6**).

Unlike NSAIDs, corticosteroids act on both cyclooxygenase and lipooxygenase pathways; hence, it is presumed to be superior to NSAIDs in controlling postoperative inflammation. Corticosteroids can be used in different ways: topical, periocular, or intravitreal. Intravitreal triamcinolone and dexamethasone implant (OZURDEX®; Abbvie) have been reported to be effective in the treatment of CME [60].

Antivascular endothelial growth factor (Anti-VEGF) plays a major role in inhibition of angiogenesis, inflammation, and capillary permeability. It is used as the first line in treating CME secondary to various vascular pathologies (e.g., diabetic macular edema, retinal vein occlusion, and choroidal neovascular membranes) that are well-established. However, its role in the treatment of CME following cataract surgery remains unclear [56].

7. Progression of diabetic retinopathy after cataract surgery

Diabetes mellitus (DM) is a known risk factor for developing early cataract, including younger age groups. Factors that may influence the progression of diabetic retinopathy (DR) and development of diabetic macular edema (DME) after cataract surgery include the following: the type and duration of diabetes, high level of glycated hemoglobin (HbA1c), the stage of retinopathy, pre-existing DME, and associated systemic diseases (e.g., hypertension and hyperlipidemia) [61].

The association between cataract surgery and progression of diabetic retinopathy has been highlighted by many authors [57, 62]. Some authors have reported an increase in the risk of progression after cataract surgery, whereas others concluded no significant difference and the progression of diabetic retinopathy (DR) is part of the natural course of the disease [63–65].

Evaluation and management: Surgery is the ultimate treatment for cataract. Planning early cataract surgery before progression of cataract further may limit retina visualization and optimization of the DR and/or DME treatment is important for continuity of care and better postoperative results. The advances in surgical techniques and pre- and postoperative diagnostic and pharmacological management of DR and/or DME have made cataract surgery safer and resulted in better outcomes, particularly for people with diabetes [66].

Prior to cataract surgery, patients with or without DR must undergo thorough eye evaluation, including dilated fundus examination to identify the level of DR and roll-out presence of DME.

Thereafter to address the need for any treatment of DR and/or DME prior to cataract surgery. Optimal management of DR and/or DME prior to cataract surgery contributes to better visual outcome and may reduce the progression of DR and/or DME after cataract surgery [65] (**Figure 7**).

It has been agreed upon that pre-excising DME should be optimally treated prior cataract surgery and careful monitoring postoperatively is recommended. The treatment options for pre-existing DME include the following: intravitreal anti-VEGF, intravitreal steroids injection or dexamethasone implants, and macular laser in particular for non-centrally involved DME. Each of those options have variable benefits and potential risks, and, therefore, the optimal choice for such treatment options is to be individualized and tailored based on the characteristics of the condition [67].

Patients with pre-existing active proliferative diabetic retinopathy (PDR) are more likely to progress further and might be complicated by vitreous hemorrhage and/or diabetic tractional retinal detachment. Therefore, panretinal photocoagulation (PRP) should be considered preoperatively [68]. Moreover, the use of anti-VEGF for PDR is emerging. In a recent systemic review with network meta-analysis (MMA) of randomized clinical trials (RCTs) comparing PRP versus anti-VEGF treatment alone or in

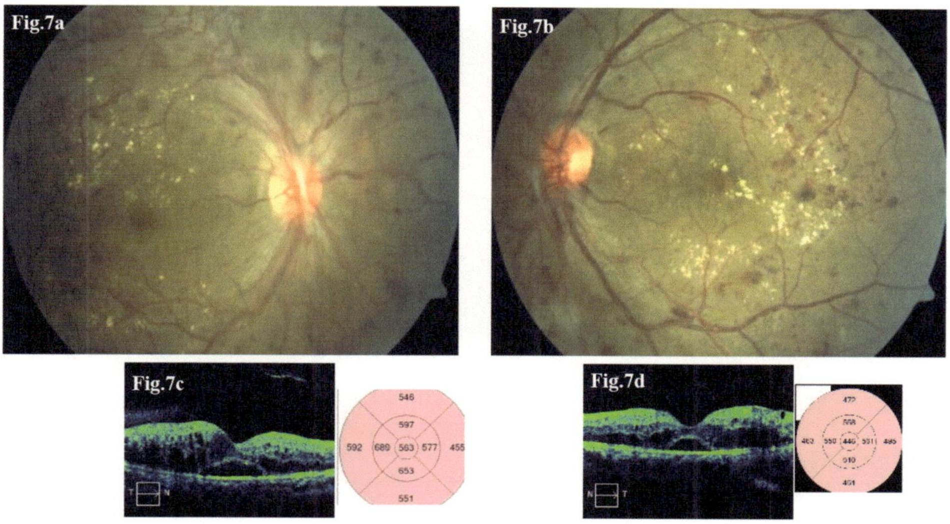

Figure 7.
Fundus photos and macula OCT showing PDR (a, b) and center-involved diabetic macular edema (c,d) in both eyes (courtesy of Dr. M. Al-Abri).

combination with PRP for PDR, it has been concluded that there is limited evidence of comparable efficacy in terms of neovascularization regression between PRP for PDR and anti-VEGF therapy alone or in combination with PRP for PDR. However, better visual outcomes were associated with anti-VEGF use [69].

8. Conclusion

In this chapter, we have discussed the most important aspects of posterior segment complications and challenges that might be encountered in the setting of cataract surgery. Though modern cataract surgery has become reasonably safe and successful as a result of the advancement in ophthalmic technology, surgical skills, and training, yet such complications might occur and, therefore, the primary surgeons and patients should be fully aware of such potential challenges and to adopt safe and evidence-based approach to overcome such challenges, which ultimately will improve the outcomes.

Acknowledgements

We would like to thank Dr. Ahmed Al-Hinai, sr. consultant VR surgeon, Sultan Qaboos University Hospital, Muscat, Sultanate of Oman, for sharing clinical photos and to thank all ophthalmic technicians in the department of ophthalmology at Sultan Qaboos University Hospital for the excellent clinical images.

Author details

Mohamed Al-Abri*, Washoo Mal and Nawal Al-Fadhil
Department of Ophthalmology, Sultan Qaboos University Hospital, Muscat, Sultanate of Oman

*Address all correspondence to: msalabri@squ.edu.om

References

[1] Desai P, Minassian D, Reidy A. National cataract surgery survey 1997-8: A report of the results of the clinical outcomes. The British Journal of Ophthalmology. 1999;**83**:1336-1340

[2] Androudi S, Brazitikos PD, Papadopoulos NT, Dereklis D, Symeon L, Stangos N. Posterior capsule rupture and vitreous loss during phacoemulsification with or without the use of an anterior chamber maintainer. Journal of Cataract and Refractive Surgery. 2004;**30**:449-452

[3] Gimbel HV, Sun R, Ferensowicz M, Anderson Penno E, Kamal A. Intraoperative management of posterior capsule tears in phacoemulsification and intraocular lens implantation. Ophthalmology. 2001;**108**:2186-2189

[4] Tan JHY, Karwatowski WSS. Phacoemulsification cataract surgery and unplanned anterior vitrectomy: Is it bad news? Eye. 2002;**16**:117-120

[5] Blomquist PH, Rugwani RM. Visual outcome after vitreous loss during cataract surgery performed by residents. Journal of Cataract and Refractive Surgery. 2002;**28**:847-852

[6] Chan FM, Mathur R, Ku JJK, Chen C, Chan S, Yong VSH, et al. Short-term outcomes in eyes with posterior capsule rupture during cataract surgery. Journal of Cataract and Refractive Surgery. 2003;**29**:537-541

[7] Cohen SM, Davis A, Cukrowski C. Cystoid macular edema after pars plana vitrectomy for retained lens fragments. Journal of Cataract and Refractive Surgery. 2006;**32**:1521-1526

[8] Chalam KV, Shah VA. Successful management of cataract surgery associated with vitreous loss with sutureless small-gauge pars plana vitrectomy. American Journal of Ophthalmology. 2004;**138**:79-84

[9] Piccone MR, Sulewski ME, Kozart DM. Uses of the sheets lens glide in contemporary cataract surgery. Journal of Cataract and Refractive Surgery. 1997;**23**:7-8

[10] Moore JK, Scott IU, Flynn HW, Smiddy WE, Murray TG, Kim JE, et al. Retinal detachment in eyes undergoing pars plana vitrectomy for removal of retained lens fragments. Ophthalmology. 2003;**110**:709-713

[11] Aaberg TM, Rubsamen PE, Flynn HW, Chang S, Mieler WF, Smiddy WE. Giant retinal tear as a complication of attempted removal of intravitreal lens fragments during cataract surgery. American Journal of Ophthalmology. 1997;**124**:222-226

[12] Mantopoulos D, Hariprasad SM, Fine HF. Suprachoroidal hemorrhage: Risk factors and diagnostic and treatment options. Ophthalmic Surgery, Lasers & Imaging Retina. 2019;**50**(11):670-674

[13] Laube T, Brockmann C, Bornfeld N. Massive suprachoroidal hemorrhage: Surgical management and outcome. GMS Ophthalmology Cases. 2015;**5**. DOI: 10.3205/oc000032. Available from: http://www.egms.de/en/journals/oc/2015-5/oc000032.shtml

[14] Jiang H, Gao Y, Fu W, Xu H. Risk factors and treatments of Suprachoroidal Hemorrhage. BioMed Research International. 2022;**2022**:6539917

[15] Pershing S, Lum F, Hsu S, Kelly S, Chiang MF, Rich WL 3rd, et al.

Endophthalmitis after cataract surgery in the United States: A report from the intelligent research in sight registry, 2013-2017. Ophthalmology. 2020;**127**:151-158

[16] Shi SL, Yu XN, Cui YL, Zheng SF, Shentu XC. Incidence of endophthalmitis after phacoemulsification cataract surgery: A meta-analysis. International Journal of Ophthalmology. 2022;**15**(2):327-335

[17] Galvis V, Tello A, Sánchez MA, Camacho PA. Cohort study of intracameral moxifloxacin in postoperative endophthalmitis prophylaxis. Ophthalmology and Eye Diseases. 2014;**6**:1-4

[18] Chang DF, Braga-Mele R, Henderson BA, Mamalis N, Vasavada A, ASCRS Cataract Clinical Committee. Antibiotic prophylaxis of postoperative endophthalmitis after cataract surgery: Results of the 2014 ASCRS member survey. Journal of Cataract and Refractive Surgery. 2015;**41**(6):1300-1305

[19] Gentile RC, Shukla S, Shah M, Ritterband DC, Engelbert M, Davis A, et al. Microbiological spectrum and antibiotic sensitivity in endophthalmitis: A 25-year review. Ophthalmology. 2014;**121**(8):1634-1642

[20] Daien V, Papinaud L, Gillies MC, et al. Effectiveness and safety of an intracameral injection of cefuroxime for the prevention of endophthalmitis after cataract surgery with or without perioperative capsular rupture. JAMA Ophthalmology. 2016;**134**:810-816

[21] Lee AY, Akileswaran L, Tibbetts MD, Garg SJ, Van Gelder RN. Identification of torque Teno virus in culture-negative endophthalmitis by representational deep DNA sequencing. Ophthalmology. 2015;**122**(3):524-530

[22] Sandhu HS, Hajrasouliha A, Kaplan HJ, Wang W. Diagnostic utility of quantitative polymerase chain reaction versus culture in endophthalmitis and uveitis. Ocular Immunology and Inflammation. 2019;**27**(4):578-582

[23] Al-Abri M, Al-Hinai A, Al Hamar Y, Al-Abri H, Habsi AA, Al-Kaabi A, et al. Endophthalmitis in Oman: A descriptive retrospective multi-center study. Oman Journal of Ophthalmology. 2020;**13**:141-145

[24] Endophthalmitis Vitrectomy Study Group. Results of the Endophthalmitis vitrectomy study; a randomized trial of immediate vitrectomy and of intravenous antibiotics for the treatment of postoperative bacterial endophthalmitis. Archives of Ophthalmology. 1995;**113**:1479-1496

[25] Ho IV, Fernandez-Sanz G, Levasseur S, Ting E, Liew G, Playfair J, et al. Early pars plana vitrectomy for treatment of acute infective endophthalmitis. Asia-Pacific Journal of Ophthalmology (Philadelphia, Pa.). 2019;**8**(1):3-7

[26] Iu LPL, Chan HY, Li GKH, et al. Acute postoperative endophthalmitis after cataract operation: Result of early vitrectomy within 24 hours of presentation. London, England: Eye; 2022. DOI: 10.1038/s41433-022-02347-1

[27] Fliney GD et al. Trends in treatment strategies for suspected bacterial endophthalmitis. Graefe's Archive for Clinical and Experimental Ophthalmology. 2018;**256**:833-838

[28] Sridhar J, Kuriyan AE, Flynn HW, Miller D. Endophthalmitis caused by *Pseudomonas aeruginosa*: Clinical features, antibiotic susceptibilities, and treatment outcomes. Retina. 2015;**35**(6):1101-1106

[29] Maalouf F, Abdulaal M, Hamam RN. Chronic postoperative endophthalmitis: A review of clinical characteristics, microbiology, treatment strategies, and outcomes. International Journal of Inflammation. 2012;**2012**:313248. DOI: 10.1155/2012/313248

[30] Clark A, Morlet N, Ng JQ, Preen DB, Semmens JB. Whole population trends in complications of cataract surgery over 22 years in Western Australia. Ophthalmology. 2011;**118**:1055-1061

[31] Erie JC, Raecker MA, Baratz KH, Schleck CD, Burke JP, Robertson DM. Risk of retinal detachment after cataract extraction, 1980-2004: A population-based study. Ophthalmology. 2006;**113**:2026-2032

[32] Neuhann IM, Neuhann TF, Heimann H, Schmickler S, Gerl RH, Foerster MH. Retinal detachment after phacoemulsification in high myopia: Analysis of 2356 cases. Journal of Cataract and Refractive Surgery. 2008;**34**:1644-1657

[33] Bechrakis NE, Dimmer A. Rhegmatogenous retinal detachment: Epidemiology and risk factors. Der Ophthalmologe. 2018;**115**:163-178

[34] Mitry D, Charteris DG, Fleck BW, Campbell H, Singh J. The epidemiology of rhegmatogenous retinal detachment: Geographical variation and clinical associations. The British Journal of Ophthalmology. 2010;**94**:678-684

[35] Kim J, Ryu SY, Hong JH, Chung EJ. Incidence and risk factors for retinal detachment after cataract surgery in Korea: A nationwide population-based study from 2011 to 2015. Graefe's Archive for Clinical and Experimental Ophthalmology. 2019;**257**(10):2193-2202

[36] Tuft SJ, Gore DM, Bunce C, Sullivan PM, Minassian DC. Outcomes of pseudophakic retinal detachment. Acta Ophthalmologica. 2012;**90**:639-644

[37] Sheu SJ, Ger LP, Ho WL. Late increased risk of retinal detachment after cataract extraction. American Journal of Ophthalmology. 2010;**149**:113-119

[38] Daien V, Le Pape A, Heve D, Carriere I, Villain M. Incidence, risk factors, and impact of age on retinal detachment after cataract surgery in France: A national population study. Ophthalmology. 2015;**122**:2179-2185

[39] Boberg-Ans G, Villumsen J, Henning V. Retinal detachment after phacoemulsification cataract extraction. Journal of Cataract and Refractive Surgery. 2003;**29**:1333-1338

[40] Tuft SJ, Minassian D, Sullivan P. Risk factors for retinal detachment after cataract surgery: A case-control study. Ophthalmology. 2006;**113**:650-656

[41] Hilford D, Hilford M, Mathew A, Polkinghorne PJ. Posterior vitreous detachment following cataract surgery. Eye (London, England). 2009;**23**:1388-1392

[42] Ripandelli G, Coppe AM, Parisi V, Olzi D, Scassa C, ChiaravallotiA SM. Posterior vitreous detachment and retinal detachment after cataract surgery. Ophthalmology. 2007;**114**:692-697

[43] Sheu SJ, Ger LP, Chen JF. Male sex as a risk factor for pseudophakic retinal detachment after cataract extraction in Taiwanese adults. Ophthalmology. 2007;**114**:1898-1903

[44] Quek DT, Lee SY, Htoon HM, Ang CL. Pseudophakic rhegmatogenous retinal detachment in a large Asian tertiary eye Centre: A cohort study.

Clinical & Experimental Ophthalmology. 2012;**40**:e1-e7

[45] Jakobsson G, Montan P, Zetterberg M, Stenevi U, Behndig A, Lundstrom M. Capsule complication during cataract surgery: Retinal detachment after cataract surgery with capsule complication: Swedish capsule rupture study group report 4. Journal of Cataract and Refractive Surgery. 2009;**35**:1699-1705

[46] Rossetti L, Autelitano A. Cystoid macular edema following cataract surgery. Current Opinion in Ophthalmology. 2000;**11**(1):65-72

[47] Yonekawa Y, Kim IK. Pseudophakic cystoid macular edema. Current Opinion in Ophthalmology. 2012;**23**(1):26-32

[48] Flach AJ. The incidence, pathogenesis and treatment of cystoid macular edema following cataract surgery. Transactions of the American Ophthalmological Society. 1998;**96**:557-634

[49] Bélair M-L, Kim SJ, Thorne JE, Dunn JP, Kedhar SR, Brown DM, et al. Incidence of cystoid macular edema after cataract surgery in patients with and without uveitis using optical coherence tomography. American Journal of Ophthalmology. 2009;**148**(1)

[50] Hunter A, Chin EK, Telander DG. Macular edema in the era of spectral-domain optical coherence tomography. Clinical Ophthalmology. 2013;**7**:2085-2089

[51] Vukicevic M, Gin T, Al-Qureshi S. Prevalence of optical coherence tomography-diagnosed postoperative cystoid macular oedema in patients following uncomplicated phaco-emulsification cataract surgery. Clinical & Experimental Ophthalmology. 2011;**40**(3):282-287

[52] Benitah NR, Arroyo JG. Pseudophakic cystoid macular edema. International Ophthalmology Clinics. 2010;**50**(1):139-153

[53] Serra R, Sellam A, Coscas F, Bruyère E, Sieiro A, Coscas GJ, et al. Evaluation of pseudophakic cystoid macular edema using optical coherence tomography angiography. European Journal of Ophthalmology. 2018;**28**(2):234-240

[54] Loewenstein A, Zur D. Postsurgical cystoid macular edema. Macular Edema. 2010;**47**:148-159

[55] Frisina R, Pinackatt SJ, Sartore M, Monfardini A, Baldi A, Cesana BM, et al. Cystoid macular edema after pars plana vitrectomy for idiopathic epiretinal membrane. Graefe's Archive for Clinical and Experimental Ophthalmology. 2015;**253**:47-56

[56] Orski M, Gawęcki M. Current management options in Irvine–gass syndrome: A systemized review. Journal of Clinical Medicine. 2021;**10**(19):4375

[57] Jeng C-J, Hsieh Y-T, Yang C-M, Yang C-H, Lin C-L, Wang I-J. Development of diabetic retinopathy after cataract surgery. PLoS One. 2018;**13**(8)

[58] Sivaprasad S, Bunce C, Crosby-Nwaobi R. Non-steroidal anti-inflammatory agents for treating cystoid macular oedema following cataract surgery. Cochrane Database of Systematic Reviews. 2012;**2**

[59] Singh R, Alpern, Jaffe, Lehmann, Lim, Reiser, et al. Evaluation of NEPAFENAC in prevention of macular edema following cataract surgery in patients with diabetic retinopathy. Clinical Ophthalmology. 2012;**6**:1259-1269. DOI: 10.2147/OPTH.S31902

[60] Dutra Medeiros M, Navarro R, Garcia-Arumí J, Mateo C, Corcóstegui B. Dexamethasone intravitreal implant for treatment of patients with recalcitrant macular edema resulting from Irvine-Gass syndrome. Investigative Opthalmology & Visual Science. 2013;**54**(5):3320

[61] Sayin N, Kara N, Pekel G, Altinkaynak H. Authors' response. Indian Journal of Ophthalmology. 2015;**63**(12):930

[62] Pollreisz A, Schmidt-Erfurth U. Diabetic cataract—Pathogenesis, epidemiology and treatment. Journal of Ophthalmology. 2010;**2010**:608751. DOI: 10.1155/2010/608751

[63] Tham Y-C, Liu L, Rim TH, Zhang L, Majithia S, Chee ML, et al. Association of cataract surgery with risk of diabetic retinopathy among Asian participants in the Singapore epidemiology of eye diseases study. JAMA Network Open. 2020;**3**(6)

[64] Krepler K, Biowski R, Schrey S, Jandrasits K, Wedrich A. Cataract surgery in patients with diabetic retinopathy: Visual outcome, progression of diabetic retinopathy, and incidence of diabetic macular oedema. Graefe's Archive for Clinical and Experimental Ophthalmology. 2002;**240**(9):735-738

[65] Chan LK, Lin SS, Chan F, Ng DS-C. Optimizing treatment for diabetic macular edema during cataract surgery. Frontiers in Endocrinology. 2023;**14**:1106706. DOI: 10.3389/fendo.2023.1106706

[66] Bixler J. Cataracts and their treatment in people with diabetes. ADA Clinical Compendia. 2019;**2019**(1):6-10

[67] Royle P, Mistry H, Auguste P, Shyangdan D, Freeman K, Lois N, et al. Pan-retinal photocoagulation and other forms of laser treatment and drug therapies for non-proliferative diabetic retinopathy: Systematic review and economic evaluation. Health Technology Assessment (Winchester, England). 2015;**19**(51):v-xxviii

[68] Fallico M, Maugeri A, Lotery A, Longo A, Bonfiglio V, Russo A, et al. Intravitreal anti-vascular endothelial growth factors, panretinal photocoagulation and combined treatment for proliferative diabetic retinopathy: A systematic review and network meta-analysis. Acta Ophthalmologica. 2021;**99**(6):e795-e805

[69] Zhao LQ, Cheng JW. A systematic review and meta-analysis of clinical outcomes of intravitreal anti-VEGF agent treatment immediately after cataract surgery for patients with diabetic retinopathy. Journal of Ophthalmology. 2019;**2019**